OXFORD MEDICAL PUBLICATIONS

Diagnostic E.N.T.

Diagnostic E.N.T.

G.D.L. SMYTH

D.Sc., M.Ch.(Hons), M.D., F.R.C.S., F.R.C.S. (I), D.L.O.
Eye and Ear Clinic,
Royal Victoria Hospital,
Belfast, Northern Ireland

OXFORD
OXFORD UNIVERSITY PRESS
NEW YORK TORONTO
1978

Oxford University Press, Walton Street, Oxford OX2 6DP

OXFORD LONDON GLASGOW NEW YORK
TORONTO MELBOURNE WELLINGTON CAPE TOWN
IBADAN NAIROBI DAR ES SALAAM LUSAKA ADDIS ABABA
KUALA LUMPUR SINGAPORE JAKARTA HONG KONG TOKYO
DELHI BOMBAY CALCUTTA MADRAS KARACHI

British Library Cataloguing in Publication Date

Smyth, G D L
   Diagnostic ENT. — (Oxford medical publications).
   1. Otolaryngology — Diagnosis
   I. Title II. Series
   616.2'1'025   RF48   77-30246

ISBN 0-19-261133-X

*Type set in Oxford by Oxprint Limited
Printed in Great Britain
by J.W. Arrowsmith Ltd., Bristol*

Preface

In the teaching of undergraduate medicine, too frequently the diseases of the ear, nose, and throat receive only superficial attention. The reasons for this lack lie partly in medical politics, partly in the inaccessibility of the relevant organs, and partly in the attitudes of specialists in this field. But it is certainly true that soon after qualification many doctors sorely regret their ignorance of a commonly occurring group of disease with which they will continue to be confronted throughout their careers.

Perhaps the most serious single educational deficiency for medical students studying ENT is the lack of a concise text which, avoiding irrelevancies such as surgical technique, firmly concentrates on the real basis of otorhinolaryngology, which is problem-solving.

This small book does away with some of the mystique of the headlamp, the laryngeal mirror, and the operating microscope, which are inappropriate to the average doctor. Instead it seeks to emphasize the fact that patients present themselves with symptoms, not diseases, and to explain how any doctor can combine the observations he makes using a simple otoscope and spatula with his general observation of the patient, and the answers he receives to a few well-planned questions. From that point he can either continue treatment himself or he can refer his patient to an appropriate clinic for more specialized treatment — either way the problem may then be solved.

I owe a considerable debt to those sources of fundamental knowledge to which I have frequently referred. In particular, these are the texts of Adam Politzer, Sir Charles Ballance, Chavalier Jackson, St. Clair Thompson, H. Kobrak, Hollowell Davis, and A. Tumarkin.

I hope that my friends and colleagues, especially John Ballantyne, George Blair, Douglas Bryce, Desmond Dawes, Derek Gordon, William House, David Lim, Brian McCabe, Harold Schuknecht, George Shambaugh, John Shea, Henry Shaw, Philip Stell, Stuart Stronge, and Juergen Tonndorf, will recognize and take pleasure in their obvious influence. In particular, I wish to thank David Austin and Jacob Sade for the many pearls of wisdom they have offered me over the years.

Finally, I would pay tribute to the work of the late Kennedy Hunter who did so much to create the Eye & Ear Clinic of the Royal Victoria Hospital, Belfast.

Belfast   G.D.L.S.
March 1977

Acknowledgements

My sincere thanks are due to:

my colleagues, Robert McCrea, Walter Doyle-Kelly, and Lindsay Slack for their helpful criticisms;

Miss Helen McIlhenney whose beautiful illustrations do much to explain what I tried to say with words;

Mr R.G. Wood without whose patient co-operation and professionalism the results of my work would have been much less presentable; and

Miss May Weller who typed the manuscript.

Contents

The ear

1. Anatomy and physiology

The ear is a highly specialized sensory organ designed (1) to collect and amplify sound converting it into electrical energy which is finally distributed to the auditory centres of the temporal cortex, and (2) to inform the organism about alternations in spatial relationship to its environment.

THE AUDITORY ORGAN (Fig. 1)

The collecting apparatus comprises the auricle and external auditory meatus, a medically directed tube about 25 mm long, whose outer one-third is supported by cartilage continuous with the auricle and whose inner two-thirds are surrounded by the bony tympanic plate on three aspects and roofed by the squama temporalis. The meatus is lined by keratinizing squamous epithelium, associated with

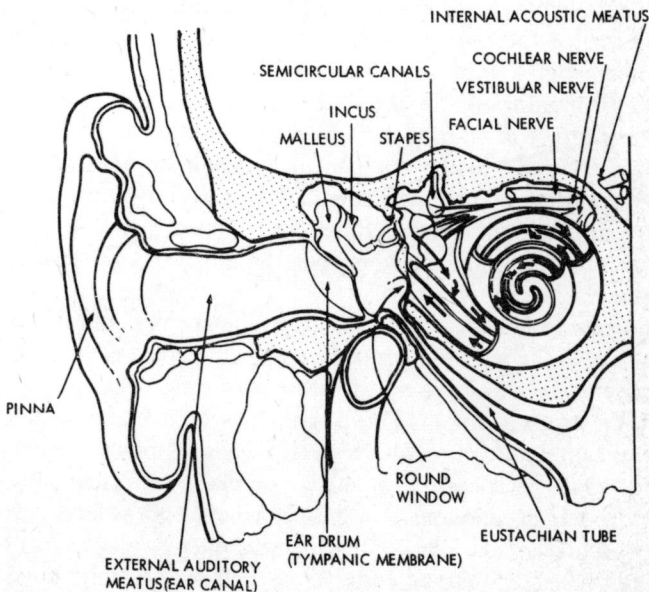

Fig. 1. General anatomy of the outer, middle, and inner ear showing the route of energy transference from the stapes footplate through the cochlea to the round window. (After Netter, F. (1962). *Ciba clin. Symp.* **14**, No. 2.)

ceruminous glands in the outer half. The health of the meatal skin depends upon a transport system whereby epithelial cells continuously move outwards from the centre of the tympanic membrane, carrying keratin and ceruminous secretion laterally along the meatus at a rate of about 30 mm per year.

The amplifying apparatus consists of the tympanum and its contents, the ossicles. The tympanum is roughly cuboidal but is indented from its lateral aspect where the three-layered tympanic membrane consisting of squamous epithelium, fibrous tissue, and mucous membrane, forms an inwardly directed cone comprising about one-half of its outer wall. The ossicles, malleus, incus, and stapes form a chain for energy transmission between the tympanic membrane and the oval window through which sound energy reaches the cochlea. Extensions of the tympanum extend posteriorly to form the mastoid air cell system and anteriorly to communicate with the nasopharynx through the Eustachian tube, through which the tympanic air pressure is regulated. The tympanum and its contents are lined by cuboidal epithelium which becomes a ciliated mucosa near the orifice of the Eustachian tube. The basis of the tympanic transformer system comprises energy coupling over a wide area between the malleus handle and the tympanic membrane, the lever ratio of the ossicular chain, and the focusing effect of transmission from the wide surface of the tympanic membrane to the comparatively small surface area of the stapes footplate. This mechanical advantage provides a means of overcoming the impedence inherent in the transmission of sound energy across the interface between the air of the tympanum and the fluid of the labyrinth.

The conversion apparatus conists of the cochlea and its central connections through the auditory nerve, the cochlear nuclei, and the ascending pathways along the second order neurones to the auditory cortex (Fig. 2). The cochlea is a coiled tube within the petrous bone which provides a system whereby physical energy is converted to electrical energy and is essentially a two-compartment structure which functions as a battery whose energy source is the stria vascularis (Fig. 3). A membranous duct (scala media) containing positively charged endolymph, rich in potassium ions, has above and below in the scala vestibuli and tympani the relatively less positively charged perilymph, rich in sodium. A continuous flow of potassium ions across the scala media to the organ of Corti (whose hair cells carry a negative charge) causes the release of transmitter substance at the synapses located at the base of the hair cells. This flow is varied by changes in electrical resistance brought about by alterations in the physical relationship between the cilia of the hair cells and the tectorial membrane which overlies them.

The relationship between cilia and tectorial membrane and thus the electrical resistance is governed by movements of the basement membrane to which the hair cells are firmly attached by their supporting cells (Fig. 4). In turn, the basement membrane is driven by a travelling wave which originates at the oval window and is due to the inward displacement of the stapes footplates — the piston end of the amplifying apparatus — resulting in a movement of the endolymph and perilymph which finally moves the round window membrane outwards (Fig. 5). By virtue of graduated variations in length and tension of its fibres, the basement membrane performs as a

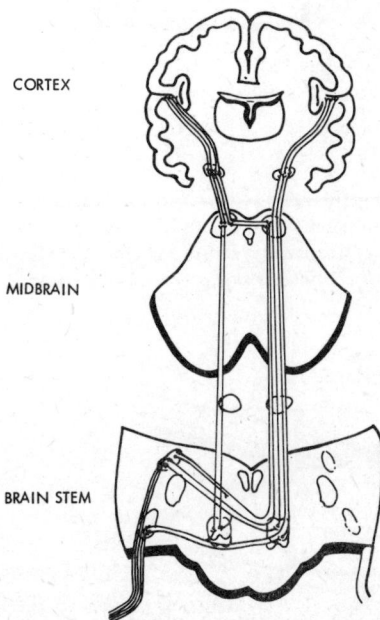

CORTEX

MIDBRAIN

BRAIN STEM

Fig. 2. The afferent pathways from the auditory neurone cells through the cochlear nuclei, which are situated in the brain stem, through the midbrain to the auditory centre located predominantly in the contralateral temporal lobe.

tuned resonator, so that it responds maximally to high-frequency stimuli as its basal end and maximally to low-frequency stimuli at its apical end with varied areas of response distributed in between.

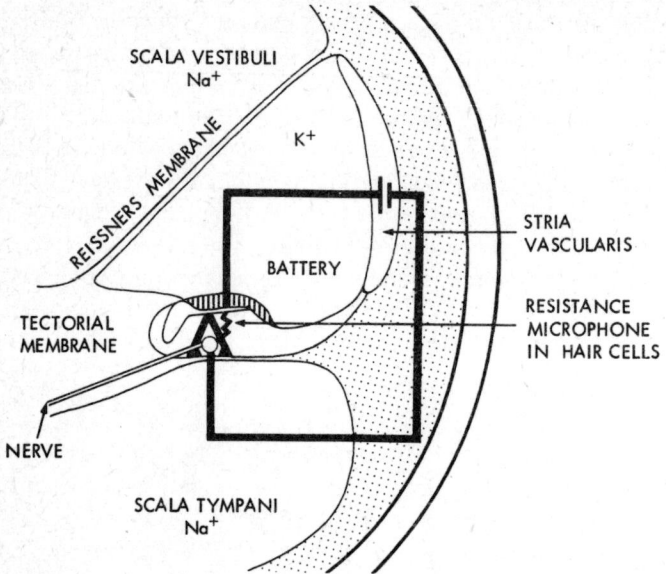

Fig. 3. Model for the generation of cochlear electrical potential. The hair cells are assumed to act as a variable resistance and thus modulate the current through the nerve endings. This is essentially a battery system (after Davis (1956). In *Physiological triggers and discontinuous rate processes.* American Physiological Society, Washington).

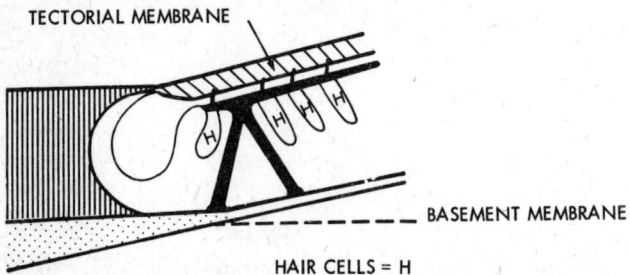

Fig. 4. Movement of the organ of Corti and the tectorial membrane, based on description by von Bekesy. The shearing action between these two stiff structures bends or shears the hairs of the hair cells (after Davis (1956); see caption to Fig. 3).

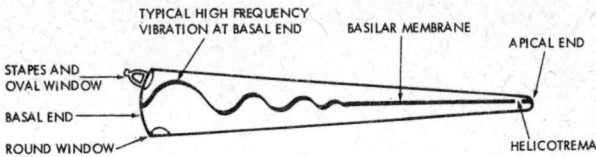

Fig. 5.

THE EQUILIBRATORY ORGAN

The equilibratory organ, or vestibule, consists of

(1) three semicircular canals set in planes roughly at right angles to each other which signal changes in angular acceleration, i.e. turning movements, and

(2) the utricle continuously providing evidence about the head's position in space and registering alterations in linear acceleration in relation to gravity, i.e. nodding and tilting movements.

Each **semicircular canal** is an osseous tube containing perilymph which in turn surrounds a membranous tube carrying endolymph. One end of each membranous tube is expanded to form an ampulla which contains the sensory apparatus of the system. This consists of a number of hair cells, grouped together to form a basally hinged flange (crista) which is deflected by currents created by the flow of endolymph which occurs during positional changes in the plane of the canal (Fig. 6). Distortion of the hair cells alters the electrical resistance of the hair cell membrane resulting in the release of transmitter substance at the synapse situated at the hair cell base and thus firing the first-order neurone. The resultant stimulus is then carried by the fibres of the vestibular branch of the eighth nerve to the vestibular nuclei situated in the brain stem.

The utricle contains the macula, a broadly based mass of hair cells attached to the wall of the membranous duct where this duct forms a chamber with which the semicircular canals communicate at their anterior ends. This membranous chamber — the utricle — lies in the posterior part of the vestibule of the inner ear and communicates anteriorly through another chamber, the saccule, whose function is not known, with the cochlear duct. Attached to the cilia of the utriclar cells are small calcified particles (statoconia) which, because of their mass being greater than that of the hair cells and thus subject to relative inertia, cause distortion of the hair cell during tilting movements (Fig. 7). This distortion alters the

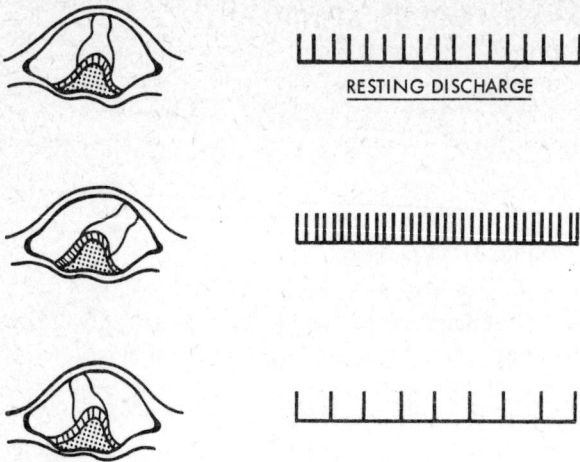

Fig. 6. At rest there is a constant discharge. This discharge increases during rotation in one direction and decreases when the direction of movement is reversed. (By permission of McCabe, B.F.)

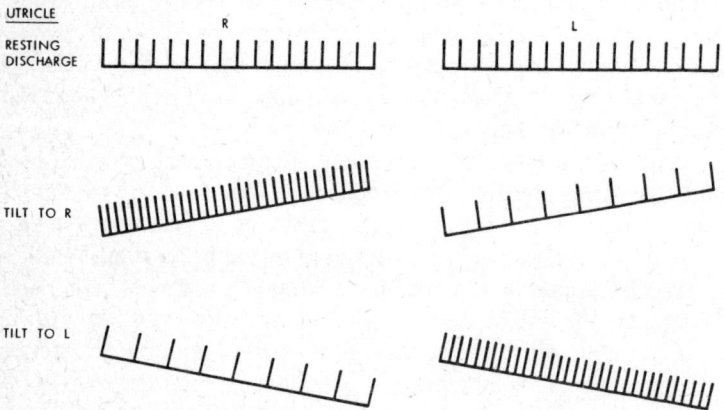

Fig. 7. During tilting, the electrical output of one utricle is the complement of the other. (By permission of McCabe, B.F.)

resistance of the hair cell; current flows, and transmitter substance is released to trigger the first-order neurone, which connects through the vestibular nerve with the vestibular nuclei.

Maintaining balance: the computer analogy

In a consideration of how the organism maintains its relationship to the environment the analogy of a computer is useful, on the basis of its input, its central analysis, and its output (Fig. 8(a) and (b)). The input is derived from visual and musculo-skeletal sources

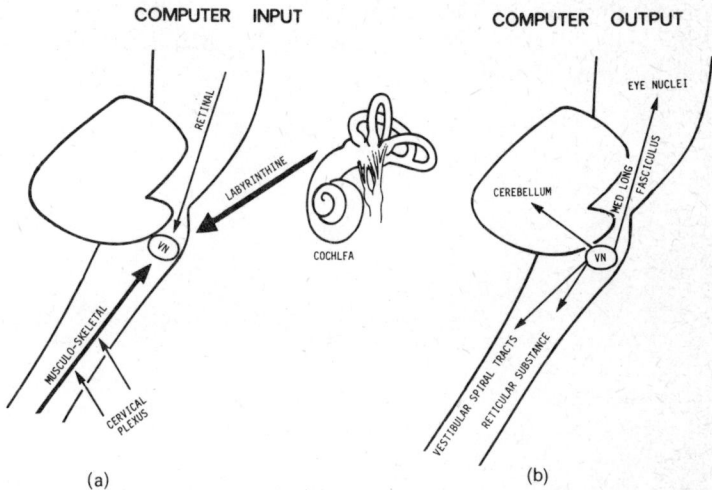

Fig. 8.

and, most importantly, from the labyrinth. This information is analysed in the brain stem mostly by the vestibular nuclei and the reticular substance and the output is distributed to those parts of the body whose role is to maintain the relationship of the organism to its environment. At rest, both labyrinths have a constant and equal discharge.

If angular acceleration or changes in linear acceleration relative to the force of gravity are imposed upon the organism then the electrical balance between the input from each labyrinth is altered. One labyrinth increases, while the other labyrinth decreases its input proportionately, maintaining throughout a constant total overall level of labyrinthine input. These data are analysed in the brain stem and correlated with data from other sources so that the resultant information can be distributed

(1) to the sensory cortex stating the extent, rate, and duration of movement,

(2) to the eye nuclei causing deviation of the eyes to maintain the last field of gaze,

(3) to the alimentary canal, if the motion is violent enough, to reduce the degree of peristalsis and close the sphincters, and

(4) finally via the motor cortex to the muscles of the limbs and spinal column in order to alert them to the state of change which is about to occur. This is the normal situation, and its basis, which is fundamental to success is the correct function of all three elements of the 'computer'.

2. Earache

Earache is usually due to inflammation of the outer or middle ear. However, it should be remembered that because the ear has several sources of sensory innervation, pain can also be referred from the pharynx, larynx, maxilla, masticatory apparatus, and upper cervical spine. Hence, the diagnosis may often require a complete examination of the head and neck.

CAUSES IN THE OUTER EAR
The pinna

1. Traumatic causes

Signs and symptoms. Painful and tender swelling of the auricle following a recent injury.

Treatment. If swelling is fluctuant, aspiration, which may require several repetitions, combined with pressure dressing, until the normal contour is restored.

Complications.
(a) Infection progressing to perichondritis.
(b) Permanent deformity (cauliflower ear) due to fibrous contracture following inadequate or delayed treatment.

2. Inflammatory causes

Signs and symptoms. The four cardinal signs of inflammation (swelling, redness, tenderness, and heat) often accompanied by pyrexia. Furunculosis (much less often herpes oticus and erysipelas) is the predominant cause. Inflammation may also arise as a complication of trauma.

Treatment.
(a) Analgesics combined with an antibiotic appropriate to staphylococcus or streptococcal infections and local heat.
(b) Aspiration should an abscess develop.

Complications. Permanent deformity due to cartilage necrosis.

The external auditory meatus

1. *Traumatic causes*

Signs and symptoms. Pain may result from the patient's own attempts to remove wax or relieve itch using a hair clip or other such instrument. Pain may also be due to roughly performed syringing for wax. Otoscopy will reveal bruising or laceration of the meatal skin and there may be bleeding.

Treatment. Oral analgesics, if required, combined with sedative drops such as Auralgicin (ephedrine hydrochloride, benzocaine, chlorbutol, potassium hydroxyquinoline sulphate, phenazone, glycerin) are usually adequate. If there is also evidence of inflammation, then the treatment is that of acute external otitis (see below).

2. *Inflammatory causes*

Signs and symptoms. Earache with tenderness on tragal pressure or movement of the pinna. Localized or generalized swelling of the meatal skin often prevents insertion of an aural speculum. Swelling can be either localized as a small boil (furuncle) (Fig. 9),

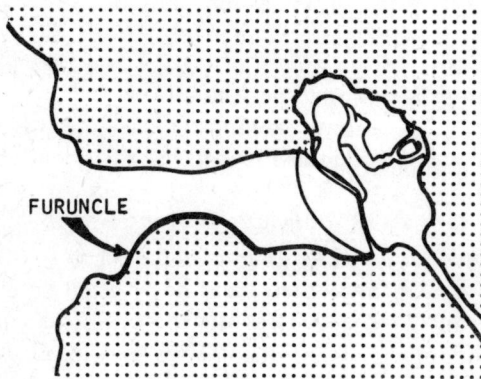

FURUNCLE

Fig. 9.

or involve the outer two-thirds of the ear canal. The organism in furunculosis is *Staphylococcus aureus,* but in the generalized form of external otitis, *Proteus, Pyocyaneus,* and coliform bacteria predominate. In some cases, fungi (yeasts and aspergilli) are initial pathogens or occur secondarily due to prolonged topical use of antibiotic and steroid drugs. A history of water in the ear from hair-washing, swimming, or trauma from hair clips, etc. is common in both types of external otitis. Myringitis bullosa, an occasional complication of viral upper respiratory infection, gives rise to haemorrhagic blebs on the lateral aspect of the tympanic membrane. Differentiation from acute middle ear infection can be difficult, and is usually made retrospectively on the basis of rapid recovery and lack of conductive hearing loss.

Treatment.
(a) Analgesics combined with appropriate broad-spectrum antibiotic in adequate dosage. Local application of heat. Whenever possible, cultura of discharge should be performed at the onset of treatment.
(b) Twice daily insertion of half-inch gauze strips soaked in glycerine and icthammol during the stage of acute swelling (for hygroscopic effect). Once the lumen of the ear canal begins to be re-established continue treatment with Genticin (gentamycin) or Otosporin (polymyxin B sulphate, neomycin sulphate, hydrocortisone) drops three times daily for several days after the subsidence of pain, followed by boric acid and spirit drops twice daily for a week (to lessen risks of recurrance).
(c) Note that if the initial swab report indicates fungal infection or if this is suspected because the secretion has a yeasty odour, antibiotic therapy is contraindicated and should be replaced forthwith by the topical use of a potent antifungal agent such as Hibitane (chlorhexidine gluconate) or Nystatin. (The growth rates of *Candida albicans* and *Aspergillus niger* are enormously increased by the topical use of steroid and broad-spectrum antibiotic.)

Complications.
1. Involvement of pre- and postaural glands causing swelling with possible abscess formation. The occurrence of postaural swelling should raise the question of acute mastoid disease. This may be difficult to eliminate from the differential diagnosis because
    (a) meatal narrowing restricts inspection of the tympanic membrane so that the diagnostic signs of otitis media which must co-exist with mastoiditis cannot be properly looked for, and
    (b) meatal swelling can also occur in mastoiditis due to osteitis, but note that this commences in the inner one-third of the ear canal, most often in the postero-superior quadrant.

Note that in superficial infections, obliteration of the postaural groove is common, whereas the groove is preserved when inflammation is subperiosteal as in acute mastoiditis.

3. *Neoplastic causes*

Signs and symptoms. Persistent discomfort often increasing to acute pain accompanied by purulent and eventually blood-stained discharge. Because both symptoms may respond temporarily to the standard treatment of inflammatory external otitis, all relapses should be regarded with suspicion. The lesion is granular or ulcerated and the diagnosis confirmed only by biopsy. Early middle ear involvement with facial paresis is common.

Treatment. Surgical excision combined with radiotherapy.

CAUSES IN THE MIDDLE EAR

1. Trauma

Most injuries of the middle ear causing pain involve only the tympanic membrane. They are caused by a sudden increase in intrameatal pressure, either from a physical blow, as occurs in body-contact sports and marital disputes, or because of bomb blast. (When a defect of the tympanic membrane is detected *following* ear syringing for wax this is usually because an abnormality of the tympanic membrane existed *before* syringing and was not anticipated through inadequate history-making regarding prior ear symptoms. When a history of a perforation or of otorrhoea is obtained, the patient should be referred to an otologist so that wax can be removed with a wax hook or by suction with, if necessary, the asisstance of magnification.)

Signs and symptoms. Pain is usually accompanied by hearing loss which is related both to the size of the tympanic membrane defect and any concussive effect on the cochlea.

Otoscopy reveals either dark coloration of the tympanic membrane due to blood in the middle ear, or a perforation whose dimensions vary from a small slit to a large, oval or kidney-shaped defect, whose edge is ragged and not smooth as in chronic suppurative otitis media. If the injury is recent there may be blood in the ear canal.

Treatment. This is primarily one of watchful expectancy because most small and many large perforations in this category will heal provided the ear is kept dry. There is no evidence that ear drops improve the prognosis and indeed they may even be harmful. Nose-blowing and sneezing against occluded nostrils should be avoided as far as possible. Discomfort is rarely acute but oral analgesics may be useful for a short period. Blood in the middle ear will usually resolve spontaneously. Should a perforation fail to heal in one month, then reference to an otologist is necessary so that treatment to close the perforation by chemical cautery or myringoplasty, as indicated, can be arranged.

Pain with bleeding from rupture of the tympanic membrane not infrequently complicates fracture of the temporal bone. Conductive and perceptive hearing loss with or without facial paresis and vertigo are commonly present and all such patients require urgent specialist otological consultation.

2. Acute inflammation of the middle ear

Acute suppurative otitis media (ASOM) arises most frequently as a complication of infection of the upper respiratory tract during the first decade of life.

Signs and symptoms. These vary with the duration of the condition. At the onset, otoscopy reveals injection of the vessels around the periphery of the tympanic membrane and along the malleus handle (Fig. 10). At this stage the patient will experience growing discomfort, 'blockage', and hearing loss. As the inflammatory process develops, the normal pearl-grey appearance of the tympanic membrane will change progressively through crimson to dusky purple.

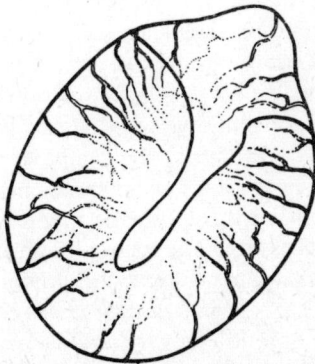

Fig. 10. Appearance of the TM in the early stages of ASOM.

As this occurs the principle landmark, the malleus handle, will become less easily seen and as the volume of purulent fluid within the middle ear space increases the *posterior* part of the tympanic membrane will bulge so as to appear much nearer than usual to the eye of the examiner. Simultaneously, the angle between the postero-superior meatal wall and the tympanic membrane will become increasingly ill-defined. As distension of the tympanic membrane proceeds, so does necrosis, leading to perforation followed by the escape of purulent discharge from the middle ear. From this stage pain and pyrexia usually begin to diminish until the disease process ultimately resolves.

Treatment. Although in many cases ASOM will settle spontaneously, to spare the patient unnecessary suffering and to avoid complications, treatment should be started as quickly as possible. This consists of:

(a) Oral analgesics and antipyretic drugs (aspirin).

(b) Oral antibiotics in adequate amounts. Unless there is evidence from bacteriological culture to the contrary, ampicillin 250–500 mg (as appropriate to body weight) six-hourly for one week is given while progress is satisfactory. (The importance of the duration of antibiotic therapy will be explained in the section on complications.)

(c) If pain and fever have not responded by 24 hours after the onset of treatment or there is other evidence that the inflammatory process is advancing then hospital admission will be necessary so that the bulging tympanic membrane can be incised under general anaesthesia (paracentesis). Failure to observe this rule is responsible for many of the complications of ASOM. For example (i) the tympanic membrane will heal more rapidly should it be incised before a large part of its substance has become necrotic, and (ii) paracentesis will allow drainage of pus from a closed space and reduce the incidence of mastoid or intracranial involvement.

(d) It cannot be over-emphasized that ear drops *do not* assist in the resolution of ASOM while the tympanic membrane is intact and their presence in the ear canal renders more difficult the task of visual assessment of the tympanic membrane should hospital referral become necessary. The value of ear drops after the onset of a perforation will depend upon the pressure of inflammatory fluid in the middle ear — when discharge has ceased to be pulsatile then drops may be able to enter the middle ear space and assist in the process of healing

It should be noted that in ASOM, as in *all* other forms of middle ear infection, concurrent nasal sinus, and nasopharyngeal infections frequently play an important role and these conditions must also be treated appropriately if a successful outcome of the total illness is to be achieved.

3. Acute mastoiditis

This occurs as an extension of ASOM when treatment has been inadequate, or because of unusual virulence of the causative organism, defective immunity, or debility on the part of the patient.

Signs and symptoms. In general these consist of an intensification of those already present. Pyrexia may reach 38.9–40 °C (102–104 °F), and pain becomes deep-seated and more extensive in its distribution, involving particularly the mastoid area. Tenderness over the mastoid antrum (i.e. 10–20 mm directly posterior to the upper edge of the meatus) and tenderness at the mastoid tip with 'guarding' spasm of the attached head of the ipsilateral as compared to the contralateral sternomastoid strongly support the diagnosis of mastoiditis.

On otoscopy, the postero-superior quadrant of the inner one-third of the ear canal will frequently be seen to be swollen and, as a rule, profuse purulent discharge pulsates through a perforated area of the tympanic membrane. However, it should be noted that discharge is not a necessity for the diagnosis of acute mastoiditis. This is either because in some cases mucosal swelling in the narrow passage connecting the middle ear and mastoid system causes an obstruction to drainage and prevents the escape of pus from the mastoid cells or because the tympanic membrane has not yet perforated.

Treatment. In the early stages this should be as described for ASOM, except that antibiotic should be started by the intramuscular route. Paracentesis of the tympanic membrane should be carried out if drainage through a perforation has not already begun.

Failure to respond in terms of improvement in signs and symptoms, especially with the development of postaural oedema, indicates an urgent need for drainage of the mastoid air cell system by cortical mastoidectomy (Fig. 11). In this operation, through a postaural incision, the bony cortex of the mastoid process is removed with electrically driven burs so that infected mucosa, granulations, and bone can be removed from the mastoid air cells and thus the abscess drained, all in accordance with standard surgical practice.

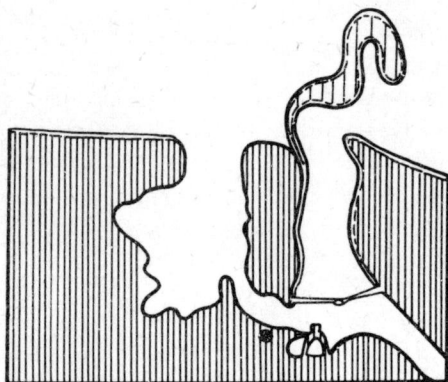

Fig. 11. In cortical mastoidectomy cortical bone overlying the mastoid cells is removed to permit the drainage of purulent secretions and the removal of granulation tissue.

Complications. These are due to extension of inflammation to the inner ear, lateral sinus, facial nerve, and intracranial spaces. The development of vertigo or evidence of decreasing cochlear function, rigors with spiking pyrexia, deep-seated parietal headache, neck stiffness, diplopia, drowsiness or coma, and failure to improve rapidly following cortical mastoidectomy must all be recognized as evidence that acute mastoid disease has now reached a highly dangerous phase which will require the combined skills of a neuro-surgical and otological team for its resolution. Prompt and free drainage of pus is the keystone of success. The aspiration of acutely life-threatening temporal lobe and cerebellar abscesses has surgical priority. As soon as the patient's condition permits, treatment of the ear condition by whichever surgical technique is required to control general mastoid infection, labyrinthitis, extradural abscess, or lateral sinus thrombophlebitis is carried out.

4. Exacerbation of chronic suppurative otitis media (CSOM)
Earache, headache, and mastoid tenderness are not normal features of the chronically infected middle ear and when this symp-

tom occurs it must be regarded as evidence of a potentially dangerous extension of the established disease.

Signs and symptoms. Mastoid tenderness, headache, and other evidence of extension of the inflammatory process, as indicated in the section concerning complications of acute mastoiditis, are all evidence of the urgent need for therapeutic action.

Treatment.

(a) Immediate broad-spectrum antibiotic such as Magnapen (ampicillin and flucloxacillin), subject to change, should the results of culture suggest otherwise, combined with analgesics and anti-pyretic drugs as appropriate.

(b) When 'medical' therapy fails to produce a rapid response (12–24 hours), then eradication of the disease process by surgical means is urgently required and is achieved by total exenteration of the diseased mucosa and bone by whatever form of mastoid operation is appropriate to the extent of the disease.

Complications. These are the same as those which occur in primary acute mastoiditis and are treated similarly.

5. Neoplasia

Although the list of neoplastic diseases involving the middle ear includes a wide range of benign and malignant conditions, including rhabdomyosarcoma, eosinophilic granuloma, leukaemia, neu-roma, glomus tympanicum and jugulare, meningioma, osteo-sarcoma, and carcinoma, earache due to neoplasia is almost invariably due to squamous or adenocarcinomata.

Signs and symptoms. Pain is usually acute and confined to the region of the ear in the early state of the disease but assumes an unremitting deep-boring nature and become less well-defined as the lesion progresses.

Although there is usually a history of long-continued aural dis-charge and hearing loss (because of undiagnosed or untreated CSOM) this is by no means always the case. Recent blood-staining of the discharge and the development of earache when there was none before are danger signs.

On examination, the findings are often not dissimilar to those in CSOM. However, the diagnosis is usually suggested by the history and by the presence of vascular granulation tissue and is based on a high index of suspicion which should always be aroused whenever CSOM *begins* to behave in an unexpected fashion. Detectable lymphatic involvement is not a feature of these conditions. The diagnosis can be confirmed only by the histological examination of tissue from the middle ear.

NON-AURAL CAUSES

The sensory innervation of both the external and middle ear is via the third division of the fifth, the seventh, ninth, and tenth cranial nerves and also the second, third, and fourth cervical spinal nerves. These nerves are also responsible for pain sensation from much of the head and neck region. Hence, pain can be referred to the ear from inflammatory and neoplastic lesions of the maxilla, nasopharynx, pharynx, larynx, tongue, tonsil, teeth, temporomandibular joint, and neck (Fig. 12).

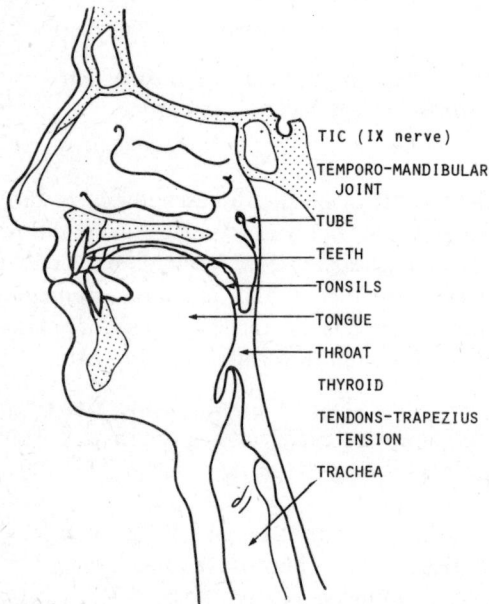

Fig. 12. The sources of pain referred to the ear. (After Tremble, G.E. (1965). *Arch Otolar.* **81**, 57-63.)

Earache in these conditions is usually less well-defined than in lesions of the ear itself and may be described by the patient as predominantly anterior or posterior to the ear. In the absence of aural findings sufficient to account for earache, the future well-being of the patient urgently demands whatever investigative procedures are necessary to detect the site and nature of the primary lesion. These will include a full ENT and dental examination supplemented, as required, by radiology and examination under general anaestheia of otherwise inaccessible regions such as the naso- and laryngopharynx.

REVISION: CAUSES OF EARACHE

For revision purposes, the causes of earache can be listed as follows:

1. Lesions affecting the **pinna**
   - (a) haematoma due to injury
   - (b) furunculosis
   - (c) herpes oticus

2. Lesions affecting the **external auditory meatus**
   - (a) instrumental trauma
   - (b) impacted wax or foreign body
   - (c) external otitis (including furunculosis)
   - (d) carcinoma
   - (e) myringitis bullosa

3. Diseases of the **middle ear**
   - (a) acute suppurative otitis media
   - (b) mastoiditis
   - (c) carcinoma

4. Referred from **elsewhere**
   - (a) masticatory apparatus
      - (i) lower molars
      - (ii) temporo-mandibular joint
   - (b) tonsil, posterior one-third tongue, and hypopharynx
      - (i) acute inflammation
      - (ii) malignancy
   - (c) cervical spine

3. Otorrhoea

Apart from cerebrospinal fluid otorrhoea, aural discharge is due to infections of the external auditory meatus or the middle ear.

EXTERNAL OTITIS
Presentation and diagnosis
If an ear has been itchy prior to discharging, then it is likely that an eczematous external otitis has become infected. Discharge is usually 'watery' at first but tends to become purulent with an unpleasant odour when the organisms responsible are *Proteus, Pyocyaneus*, or coliform. The cocha and the postaural skin crease become scaly red, and often weep.

Discomfort, pain, and tenderness will be present and the ear feels 'blocked' because of accumulated secretions in the meatus. Note that the condition is characteristically bilateral and symptoms frequently follow, or are exacerbated by water entering the meatus while swimming and hair-washing. There is a characteristic tendency to relapse.

In some patients, yeasts and aspergilli are the predominant organisms, especially if the use of antibiotic drops for an itchy eczematous ear has been prolonged. Otoscopy will reveal a white curd with a beery odour and sometimes spore heads.

ACUTE SUPPURATIVE OTITIS MEDIA
Presentation and diagnosis
If purulent and sometimes blood-stained discharge follows and is accompanied by reduction in an earache which has complicated an upper respiratory infection, and at the same time there is marked hearing loss, then the patient is most likely to be suffering from acute suppurative otitis media. This presentation differs from that of external otitis in two ways:

    (1) tenderness on moving the pinna or tragus are absent;

    (2) the severity of the illness is very much greater, the hearing loss more marked, and there is practically always a history of recent sore throat, coryza, or influenza.

CHRONIC OTITIS MEDIA

Presentation and diagnosis

When a patient reports that his permanently deaf ear has started to run again and he thinks that swimming or a cold may have been responsible, although this may be an exacerbation of external otitis, the duration of the hearing loss suggests that the patient suffers from chronic otitis media. In contrast to the watery or purulent discharge of external otitis and acute suppurative otitis media, the discharge in chronic otitis media contains mucus (mucopurulent) which gives it a 'ropy' consistency. Clinically this differs from acute suppurative otitis in that the patient does not appear to be ill and does not complain of pain or recent alteration in hearing. The presence of a tympanic membrane perforation through which the discharge can be seen to be issuing on otoscopy will confirm the diagnosis.

SKULL FRACTURE

Presentation and diagnosis

Ear discharge following head injury is diagnostic of temporal bone fracture usually with laceration of the tympanic membrane. Initially the discharge is blood-stained but becomes increasingly 'watery' and even purulent if infection supervenes, implying a grave risk of meningitis. Inspection of the tympanic membrane will reveal the exit of cerebrospinal fluid through a ragged-edged perforation.

TREATMENT

The treatment of these conditions has already been discussed.

REVISION: CAUSES OF OTORRHOEA

For revision purposes, the causes of otorrhoea can be listed as follows:

1. Causes in the **external auditory meatus**
   (a) External otitis
       (i) bacterial
       (ii) fungal
       (iii) carcinomatous

2. Causes in the **middle ear**
   (a) acute suppurative otitis media
   (b) chronic suppurative otitis media
   (c) carcinoma of the middle ear
   (d) skull fracture leading to cerebrospinal fluid otorrhoea.

4. Deafness

Deafness is classified as being (Fig. 13):

(1) **conductive,** when the cause is in the ear canal or middle ear, and

(2) **perceptive,** when the cause is in the middle ear or its central connections. This group can be subdivided into:

(a) **sensory,** when the cochlea is affected, and

(b) **neural,** when there is involvement of the neural pathways between the organ of Corti via the eighth nerve, the cochlear nuclei (CN), and the ascending tracts to the auditory cortex (AC).

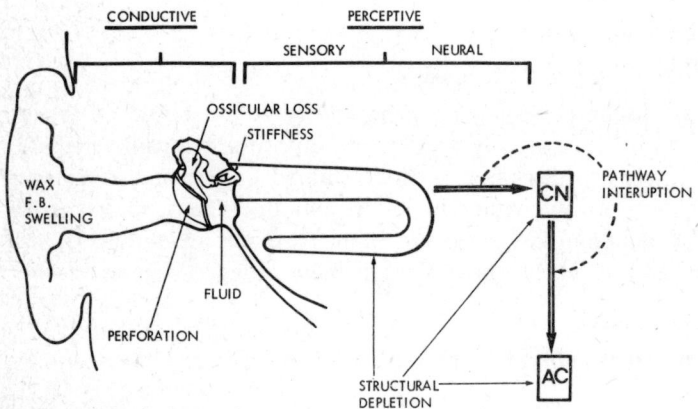

Fig. 13. Causes and types of hearing loss (F.B. = foreign body).

Diagnosis

When the onset of deafness follows a recent upper respiratory infection, often with earache, a conductive cause should be thought of first.

Perceptive hearing loss is most common in the second half of life and its nature is often indicated by concomitant tinnitus and some disturbance of balance. It should be suspected after head injury, in the young when hearing has always been deficient or where there is a family history of deafness.

In reaching a diagnosis the history as given by the patient and especially by his relatives is often most valuable. The Rinne test is useful as a simple and practical means of comparing air and bone conduction responses to a vibrating tuning fork and thus differentiating between conductive and perceptive deafness prior to full audiometric evaluation by the otologist. When the tuning fork is heard better by bone conduction in the affected ear, the cause of deafness is usually a conductive one (Rinne negative). If the tuning fork is heard better by air conduction in the deaf ear then the cause is usually a perceptive one (Rinne positive). A vibrating fork placed on the vertex (Weber test) will sound louder in the better hearing ear in perceptive deafness and louder in the worse hearing ear in conductive deafness. This test provides confirmation of the Rinne test findings.

Tuning fork tests

The value of tuning fork tests is enhanced by understanding their underlying principles.

1. *The Rinne test.* When the conduction mechanism of the middle ear is normal, not surprisingly the usual route of sound transmission is the more efficient, hence air-conducted sound appears louder than it does by bone conduction (Rinne positive). This is the case in all normal ears and in ears with hearing loss due to disease of the perceptive apparatus.

On the other hand, when defects of the conduction mechanism impair the passage of sound through the middle ear, hearing is better by bone conduction than by air conduction (Rinne negative).

2. Understanding *the Weber test* depends upon remembering that a sound stimulus from the vertex reaches both temporal bones at the same time and with equal intensity. Although most of this sound stimulates the cochlea, some of it is normally bypassed to the external ear canal via the conduction mechanism working in the reverse direction to that which is physiologically normal.

When the conduction mechanism of the middle ear is normal the Weber test is used to compare the function of one cochlea with that of the other. Consequently, the loudness of sound from the vertex, (a) will not be lateralized when both cochlea have *equal* function, be it normal or not, and (b) the sound will be lateralized, i.e. heard more loudly, by the ear whose cochlea is functionally better than the other.

When the conduction mechanism of the middle ear is not normal, then the Weber test response augments the information provided by the Rinne test. In this case, unidirectional obstruction of the bypass provided by the ossicular chain and tympanic membrane causes the stimulus to appear louder in the conductively deafened ear by

(1) preventing the escape of energy away from the cochlea, and
(2) eliminating the masking effect of environmental noise.

The causes and treatment of conductive and perceptive deafness can be classified most conveniently under the headings genetic, traumatic, neoplastic, and 'others'.

CONDUCTIVE DEAFNESS

Genetic causes

The commonest form is otosclerosis in which hardness of hearing rarely begins before the twenties. In contrast to genetic perceptive deafness, genetic conductive hearing loss in general is most rare in the first two decades. In otosclerosis, the tympanic membrane appears normal and the Rinne test is negative. Deafness is frequently bilateral, affects females twice as often as males, and is familial, the disease being transmitted as an autosomal dominant characteristic. Hearing impairment is due to abnormal bone-formation around the stapes which prevents the transmission of sound between the middle and inner ears. Sound transmission can be assisted by amplification from a hearing aid or by an operation to replace the stapes by a plastic prosthesis (stapedectomy) (Fig. 14).

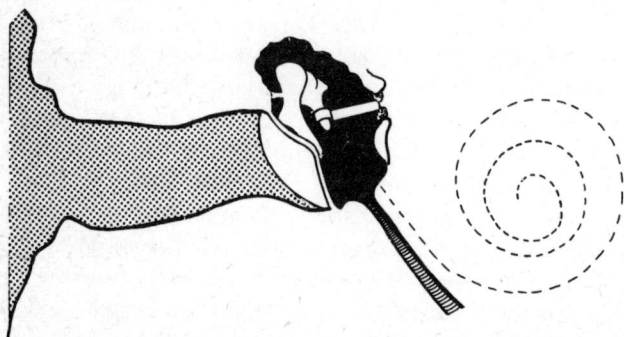

Fig. 14. Stapedectomy. After removal of the stapes arch, the footplate is removed and a teflon prosthesis placed between the incus and the oval window where it is surrounded by pieces of gelfoam or connective tissue.

Traumatic causes

There will be a history of injury, either from a foreign body in the external ear canal, or from acute air-pressure changes as occur in a blow to the side of the head, or in bomb blast, or in deep-sea diving. These may rupture the tympanic membrane or dislocate one of the ossicles. Apart from deafness, or a sense of fullness in the ear, the patient may complain of tinnitus and bleeding from the ear. Examination will usually reveal blood in the meatus and contusion of the tympanic membrane. Although the tympanic membrane is frequently perforated the exact site and dimensions of the tear are usually difficult to define owing to the presence of a clot mixed with wax and because of swelling of the tissues.

In most cases, recovery will occur spontaneously. Any attempt to clean the ear or provide topical treatment risks secondary bacterial infection. Thus drops should not be prescribed and the patient should be rigorously cautioned to prevent fluid entering the ear canal and to refrain from nose-blowing.

Although spontaneous recovery is the rule and many patients will do well without specialist examination, nevertheless, those with more than minor symptoms should be referred for otological opinion, so that (a) concomitant perceptive losses can be treated early, and (b) perforations which fail to heal can be repaired by surgical means (myringoplasty).

In cases of skull injury complicated by deafness (usually due to fracture of the temporal bone) a combined otological–neuro-surgical referral should be obtained to manage such complications as cerebrospinal fluid otorrhoea or involvement of the inner ear and facial nerve.

Inflammatory causes

Acute suppurative otitis media (ASOM)

ASOM is a frequent cause of deafness in children, whose diagnosis is usually obvious from the history of upper respiratory infection followed by earache, deafness, and discharge, etc. (The diagnosis and treatment of this condition have been dealt with in Chapter 2 on earache.)

The enormous importance of an early diagnosis and adequate treatment of ASOM cannot be over-emphasized. ASOM has always been an important threat to health. Formerly, this was mainly because of the dangers of acute mastoiditis and serious

intracranial complications such as meningitis and cerebral and cerebellar abscess, conditions whose incidence has been considerably
reduced by antibiotics. Now, the importance of ASOM lies more in
the fact that incompletely treated ASOM can lead to catarrhal
otitis media (otherwise known as secretory otitis media, serous
otitis media, and 'glue ear'), which is the commonest cause of
chronic suppurative otitis media and chronic mastoiditis.

Chronic catarrhal otitis media (CCOM)

Presentation. CCOM is a condition of the first ten years of life.
Following an upper respiratory infection in which the inflammatory
middle ear symptoms may or may not have been over-evident,
deafness will usually be noticed by the parents or teacher. The
danger is that when the condition is unilateral, with thus only a
partial defect in overall auditory capacity, there may well be some
delay in its discovery.

This danger can be largely offset by the general practitioner's
awareness that CCOM after upper respiratory infection is an ever-
present possibility and cannot be detected without examination of
the tympanic membranes two to three weeks after the event, with
supplementary audiometry, when indicated.

Diagnosis. Although there are no constant diagnostic appearances
on otoscopy, any alteration of the normal characteristics of the
tympanic membrane (TM) should be regarded as reasons for
suspecting CCOM. What is seen depends upon the duration of the
disease process.

Generally, the colour of the TM is changed from oyster grey to
dull red or yellow or alternatively assumes a darker, more opaque
appearance. The conical configuration of the TM is increased as it
becomes retracted medially and is indicated by displacement of
the malleus handle posteriorly and superiorly, coupled with
broadening and a split in, or complete loss of, the light reflex.

As the process advances, retracted areas develop posteriorly
so that the long process of the incus and stapes head appear as
lateral protrusions as the TM becomes draped around them.

Simple voice tests (a normally hearing child should have no
difficulty in repeating words whispered from 6 metres or 20 feet)
after occlusion of the opposite ear, are useful to indicate the level of
hearing. From five years and upwards, tuning fork tests can be used
to confirm the presence of a conductive loss.

Treatment. Initial treatment is best carried out at general practice level, provided that marked retraction has not yet occurred. Early cases may resolve spontaneously and the process can be assisted by the administration of (1) a *decongestant,* e.g., Actifed Compound Linctus (triprolidine hydrochlor, pseudoephedrine hydrochlor, codeine phosphate) 1·25 ml twice daily for five years and below, 2·5–5 ml twice daily for older children — the dose should be regulated to avoid side effects such as drowsiness, lack of appetite, and irritability; (2) an *antibacterial* such as Septrin Syrup (trimethoprim, sulphamethoxazole) one teaspoonful twice daily. *Both* should be given *for two weeks* and the process assisted by having the child inflate balloons by the nasal method twice daily. If, at the end of two weeks, the appearances of the TM and/or the hearing levels are not normal, the child must now be referred for otological evaluation in an ENT outpatient clinic. Management from that point onward will consist of:

1. Paracentesis (myringotomy), with suction removal of fluid and the insertion of a ventilator tube to restore the normal gaseous environment of the middle ear, so that its epithelium can revert to normal and excess mucus production cease;

2. The elimination, *when indicated,* of contributory factors such as Eustachian tube obstruction by
   (a) adenoidectomy,
   (b) reduction of the inferior tubinates by trimming and submucosal diathermy,
   (c) the erradication of sinus infection, and
   (d) treatment of nasal allergy.

Chronic suppurative otitis media (CSOM) and chronic mastoiditis
These conditions account for a large proportion of conductive deafness. Although it is true that CSOM can be the direct result of ASOM in cases where a perforation of the TM fails to heal, such an occurrence is now quite rare. In the main, CSOM is the result of unresolved catarrhal otitis media. Owing to the action of enzymes present in persistent effusions there develops an area of the TM which lacks elasticity due to loss of its fibrous tissue layer. At this stage there are three possible outcomes:

1. Nothing changes, and in later life it will be noted that there is a 'scar' of the TM which does not appear to impair hearing.

2. The week area will break down during the *next* middle ear infection (ASOM), leading to permanent perforation and the extension and perpetuation of infection throughout the tubo-tympanic cleft which we call chronic granulomatous middle ear disease (a type of CSOM).

Examination at this stage will reveal a defect of the TM of variable size, a view of the medial wall of the tympanum and possibly the ossicles (depending on the site of the defect and the survival of the ossicles), granulation tissue, and mucoid or mucopurulent discharge.

The range of appearances is extreme and varies from the simple *central* perforation, leaving a rim of remaining TM all around, with little or no mucosal or ossicular disease to generalized mucosal disease causing prolific granulomatous mucosal reaction (cholesterol granuloma) and chronic osteitis of the ossicles and the bone of the mastoid air cell system, resulting in persistent odoriferous discharge with progressive hearing loss (Fig. 15(a) and (b)).

To the examiner, even if the exact detail is not clear, *the impressions of middle ear disorder and destruction are clearly apparent* and coupled with the evidence of conductive hearing loss, are indicative of CSOM with chronic mastoiditis.

Although much can be done to alleviate the condition temporarily at general practice level, it should be emphasized that such treatment is *only palliative* and cannot be curative. Surgical treatment is necessary to remove irreversibly-infected bone and mucosa, to repair the TM defect, and reconstruct the ossicular chain. It is worth noting that preliminary therapy by toilet and irrigating drops such as Aurist acid boric is always useful to procure better operating conditions and improve the chances of surgical success by temporarily reducing inflammation.

3. The third possible outcome of CCOM also is derived from the weakened area of the tympanic membrane. As a result of persistent reduced intratympanic pressure, the traction of adhesions, and the altered direction of its growth, the weakened area of the TM recedes medially to form a retraction pocket or sac which extends progressively through the mastoid aditus, antrum, and air cell system. This sac is lined superficially by keratinizing epithelium whose product accumulates within it forming a cyst which is called cholesteatoma. Enlargement of the cholesteatoma is accompanied by erosion of bone — that of the the ossicles and that surrounding

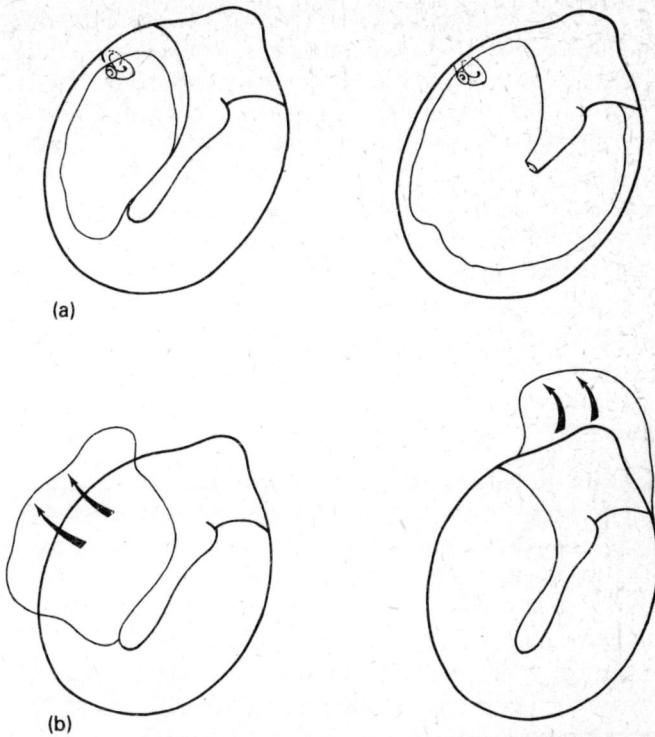

Fig. 15. (a) Perforations of the TM which result from ASOM. Note that a rim of TM survives. Untreated, this can lead to granulomatous otitis media, which is the commonest form of CSOM. (b) Defects of the TM characteristic of cholesteatomous middle ear disease. In reality these are the lateral openings of epithelial pouches containing keratin, and not perforations in the true sense. Note the absence of a continuous rim.

the mastoid air cells. Erosion is due to pressure atrophy and the destructive powers of enzymes in the accumulated keratin and the subepithelial granular layer. Thus, catarrhal otitis media can proceed to cholesteatomatous disease of the mastoid air cell system.

Untreated, cholesteatoma may, by its continued erosion, expose the dura and create a pathway for future infection which may cause facial paralysis, labyrinthitis, and meningitis or brain abscess.

During its early stages the expanding sac may bypass the ossicles and the diagnosis of cholesteatomatous ear disease is therefore based less on a history of gradually increasing hearing impairment than it is on the detection of an anatomical abnormality in the superior or the postero-superior TM. At first sight this may often appear to be a 'perforation' but in reality this is the orifice of a retracted sac arising from a previously weakened area of the TM; a retraction which in spite of its frequently innocuous appearance may extend extensively through, and even exceed the confines of, the mastoid air cell system.

It should be emphasized that cholesteatoma is not initially an acute inflammatory condition, but it will of course often become so because of secondary infection. Thus, the otoscopic appearances range from a dry postero-superior 'defect' of the TM to those of an 'acute' granular purulent process with generalized destruction of the TM, ossicles, and mastoid system (on X-ray) and evidence of the cholesteatomatous process from the presence of masses of keratin extruding out of the sac.

Treatment. In general, the aims of treatment in chronic inflammatory disease of the tubotympanic cleft, whether it be cholesteatomatous or not are (a) to eradicate irreversible disease (and thus make the ear 'safe'), and (b) to restore function.

The surgical technique is either some form of *modified radical mastoidectomy* or *tympanoplasty* (Fig. 16(a) and (b)).

In radical mastoidectomy, the osseous partition between the external auditory meatus and the mastoid air cells is removed with most of the air cell system, leaving a cavity which communicates with the exterior through the meatal orifice. The operation is 'modified' whenever the remnants of TM and ossicles can be preserved, usually in a non-functional state.

In tympanoplasty, diseased mucosa and bone are also removed extensively, but the general anatomy of the ear canal is preserved and the TM and ossicular chain reconstructed. When the extent of disease necessitates removal of the osseous canal wall then this is rebuilt with cartilage, bone, or periosteal grafts to avoid an open cavity. Although there continues to be a dispute between those who advocate modified radical mastoidectomy and those who employ tympanoplasty, there is now much evidence to support tympanoplasty as the surgical method of choice for these diseases of the tubotympanic cleft by virtue of better healing and better hearing postoperatively, and it is hoped that the problem of the 'chonic middle ear' will eventually be solved by the various forms of tympanoplasty which are currently being evolved.

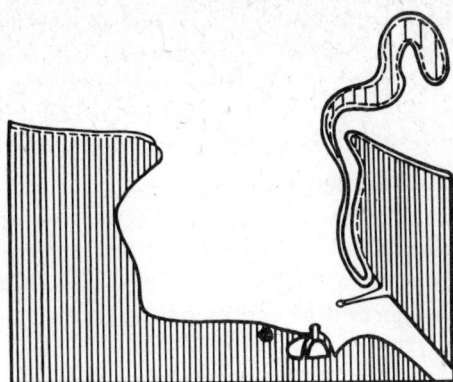

(a)

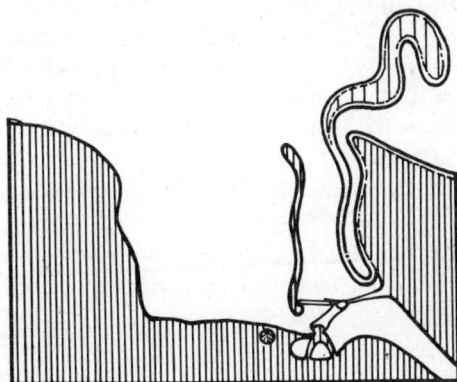

(b)

Fig. 16. (a) In modified radical mastoidectomy the walls of the mastoid air cells, granulation tissue, and remnants of the diseased ossicles are removed, so that the resulting cavity within the mastoid process can drain freely into the ear canal. Note that there is no reconstruction of the hearing mechanism. (b) In tympanoplasty the osseous ear canal is preserved in order to avoid an open cavity and the middle ear is reconstructed to improve hearing.

Whereas in CSOM without cholesteatoma, surgical therapy is *desirable* both to eradicate disease and to improve auditory function, in cholesteatomatous disease, surgery is *obligatory* in order to prevent life-threatening extension of the process. If this aim can be achieved and at the same time coupled with functional improvement then, because the condition is so often a bilateral one, much will have been done to ensure the patient's future safety and quality of life.

PERCEPTIVE HEARING LOSS

Lesions of the sensory apparatus

Sensory lesions affect the cochlea, and involve the organ of Corti, the basilar membrane, Reissner's membrane, and the stria vascularis, either singly or in combination. The causes of sensory deafness can be categorized as congenital, traumatic, inflammatory, neoplastic, and 'others'.

The history may indicate the possibility of early or late-occurring genetic cause (i.e. family history), metabolic disease, such as hypothyroidism or diabetes, trauma from bomb blast and excessive noise exposure, or infection due to lues or virus (mumps and measles).

Clinical examination usually rules out the existence of external and middle ear disease (although of course in some cases these can exist simultaneously; this is especially true of catarrhal otitis media). The affected ear is Rinne-positive but absolute bone conduction (the length of time the fork is heard on the mastoid process) is reduced.

Sensory hearing loss in childhood is usually congenital (i.e. present at birth). Much less often the loss is acquired (i.e. developed after birth).

Congenital causes

Congenital deafness may be:

(a) **Genetic,** in which case the family history of deafness, of consanguinity of parents, concurrent abnormalities in other body systems (skeletal, renal, cardiac, or ophthalmic), or the presence of an anatomic abnormality of the auricle may suggest the cause. (NB: Always look at the pinna before you examine the TM.)

(b) **Non-genetic,** in which a history of rubella during pregnancy, birth problems suggesting anoxia, and early jaundice (implying brain stem damage) may be obtained from the parents.

Diagnosis. In all children, a hearing defect should be suspected when there is failure to go through the various stages of speech development in the normal way. This failure is often associated with failure to achieve other developmental landmarks such as crawling and walking at the expected time. When a mother thinks her child is deaf she is very rarely wrong and it is unforgivable to dismiss a mother's convictions without a most careful and thorough examination of the hearing.

When this suspicion exists in the mind of the mother and is confirmed by the health visitor and/or the general practitioner, by means of hearing tests appropriate to the child's age, then immediate referral to an audiology clinic is imperative. If the diagnosis is confirmed then evaluations of the child's auditory, psychological, and educative capacities are carried out and the overall management of the child is planned from that point on.

The following milestones are achieved by the average child:

1. From soon after birth: startle response to loud sound.

2. At two months: turns head and eyes towards source of loud sound.

3. At three to four months: turns towards quieter but meaningful sounds such as spoon striking cup (indicating meal time) or mother's voice.

4. At eight months: begins babbling speech with long strings of syllables.

5. At one year: starts to pronounce individual words distinctly and knows names of objects, can obey play instructions such as 'Give me the car'.

6. At between two and three years: can respond to questions with answers in sentence form with acceptable pronunciation.

7. At four to four-and-a-half years: can be tested by audiometric techniques.

Management. The main thrust of management is to improve an already existing but defective hearing environment so that the child can establish social relationships, become educated, and eventually be able to enter society with the minimum handicap. Special teaching, especially in lip-reading, amplification with hearing aids, and parent counselling, all play important parts in the overall conduct of the situation. The object of all of these is to ensure, as early as possible, that the baby is stimulated to make the best use of its residual hearing.

Traumatic causes

Most hearing losses due to acute trauma are perceptive in type. An association between severe head injury and marked hearing loss is common — most of those exposed to bomb blast have temporary or permanent impairment of auditory function.

(a) *Head injury*. The diagnosis of cochlear damage is usually clearly indicated from the history. If the ear has bled, this suggests strongly the probability of temporal bone fracture, a diagnosis supported by concomitant facial weakness and vertigo and confirmed by X-ray. In this case, the main responsibility for patient management is neurosurgical. As a rule, the hearing loss is permanent and unresponsive to treatment. However, when fracture has not occurred and the injury is concussive, some spontaneous recovery may occur and some patients may be assisted by early treatment with steroids and vasodilators.

(b) *Bomb blast*. In this, first compressive and then rarifying pressure forces injure the organ of Corti. To some extent the effects are reversible, depending on the degree of damage and the reserve function of the ear. Deafness due to structural loss will not recover, but the recovery of metabolically deranged hair cells can be promoted after hospitalization by improving cochlear microcirculation through the use of vasodilators (Opilon 80 mg six-hourly, 5% carbon dioxide inhalations for one hour six-hourly, low molar dextran intravenously, 1 l daily) and by assisting cellular metabolism with steroids.

(c) *Noise-induced hearing loss*. This cause of deafness can be detected by the doctor, only by asking the correct questions regarding, first the type of work, the noise level (levels greater than 90 dB are extremely dangerous), the duration of exposure, etc., and, secondly, other noisy activities, use of firearms in armed forces or sport, use of noisy equipment in hobbies or amusements.

The external auditory meatus and TM are normal. The response to the usual tuning fork tests using the 512 fork is also usually normal. This is because, initially, the hearing loss affects the high-frequency response area of the cochlea, the apical turns being relatively immune. This difference in effect is illustrated dramatically in the audiometric record which shows an elevation of threshold, initially at 4000 Hz, but later involving adjacent frequencies as well: involvement which increases as exposure to sound pressure levels over 90 dB continues.

Frequently, the patient will initially complain more of tinnitus than of hearing loss. In the early stages of the process the auditory defect is reversible (temporary threshold shift) but as exposure continues, recovery becomes less possible until eventually the hair cells are irreversibly damaged.

No medical therapy has any improving effect on this problem once established but much can be done through advice and warings regarding the risks of high levels of noise at work and in sport. Further loss can be prevented by ear protection with muffs and ear plugs.

Inflammatory causes

Sensory hearing loss frequently accompanies conduction loss in ASOM, and although inner ear involvement initially is usually subliminal and does not *at the time* appear to affect auditory function, nevertheless this gradually deteriorates and the results become apparent in later life. The passage of bacterial toxins and tryptolytic enzymes through the round window membrane into the labyrinth causes hair cell death in that part of the cochlea which is specifically responsible for high-frequency reception.

Sensory hearing loss may also complicate uncontrolled chronic middle ear and mastoid infection and is the result of the passage of organisms and toxins into the inner ear through the oval or round windows, or through a pre-existing defect in the labyrinthine wall due to fracture or cholesteatomatous erosion. The result is labyrinthitis which causes total and complete loss of hearing and acute vertigo. The treatment of such a situation is based on massive antibiotic therapy (broad-spectrum, intravenously, until a bacteriological diagnosis is established) coupled with urgent surgical drainage of the labyrinth.

Most infections of the middle ear are bacterial. Such a predominance tends to diminish the recognition which is given to the very small proportion of other inflammatory forms of labyrinthitis. One of these is due to *Treponema pallidum,* and congenital lues is responsible for a particularly intractible form of sensory deafness. Because its clinical presentation is very similar to Ménière's disease (to be discussed later) the correct diagnosis is often not made while the disease is in its early still-treatable phase. A constant awareness of the possibility of congenital lues as a cause of sensory deafness; the routine performance of the fluorescent trepenoma antibody absorption test (FTA-abs.) (because of prior penicillin therapy the Wassermann is often negative); and the routine enquiry into past history to produce evidence of repeated abortions ('miscarriages'), interstitial keratitis (childhood 'eye trouble'), and similar symptoms in siblings are clearly all-important in establishing the diagnosis. Treatment over the longterm, through a combination of steroids and ampicillin (which requires frequent otologic and metabolic monitoring) can frequently prevent the progression of inevitable hearing loss to a state of 'stone-deafness'.

Viral labyrinthitis, mumps, and measles, especially in childhood, are occasionally complicated by gross or total sensory hearing loss which, if unilateral, as is fortunately usually the case, is generally detected inadvertently at some interval after the event. When the organisms of viral or bacterial meningitis pass from the internal auditory meatus along canaliculi of the eighth nerve to the labyrinth, should the patient survive his illness, hearing loss is frequently bilateral and total.

Neoplastic causes

Benign and malignant tumours in the petrous temporal bone are extremely rare causes of sensory deafness. They include eosinophilic granuloma, meningioma, congenital cholesteatoma, and neuroma of the facial nerve. Secondary spread from the middle ear of carcinoma and adenocarinoma or metastatic deposits from primary carcinoma of the bronchus, thyroid, and kidney are other rare causes of sensory hearing loss.

Otoscopic examination reveals no abnormality unless the tumour has extended to the middle ear space and the TM. Differentiation from other causes of sensory deafness is usually based on the routine tomographic radiological studies which are an essential part of *all* unilateral perceptive hearing losses.

Treatment is by surgical extirpation, combined with radiotherapy in malignant lesions, but the aim of treatment for these is largely palliative rather than curative.

Other causes

(a) *Vascular* (Fig. 17). Microcirculatory failure is responsible for most cases of sudden deafness with or without vertigo. The patient is usually in middle life and there may be evidence of generalized circulatory disease. Frequently a recent history of viral infection is obtained which, *per se,* leads to increased stickiness of the red blood corpuscles and platelets coupled with endothelial swelling which together cause a reduction in cochlear oxygen tension.

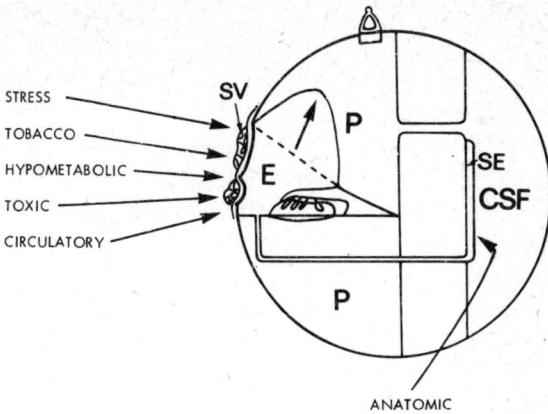

Fig. 17. The volume of endolymph (E) can be affected adversely with displacement of Reissner's membrane into the perilymphatic space (P) because of vascular factors which (a) affect the function of the stria vascularis (SV), (b) affect the absorptive function of the saccus endolymphaticus (SE), often associated with anatomical abnormalities of the endolymphatic duct. (After Lawrence, M. (1965). *Ann. Otol. Rhinol. Lar.* **74**, 489–99.)

Patients with defects in metabolism, especially diabetes, are at risk. Following fracture of the long bones, especially the femoral neck, fat emboli may cause obstruction of one or several of the small vessels of the cochlea.

Diagnosis and management depend on an awareness of the mechanisms of microcirculatory disease of the inner ear and of its importance as a forerunner of generalized vascular disease. The treatment consists of immediate attempts to increase the cochlear circulation and includes the use of vasodilators such as Opilon (thymoxamine) 80 mg six-hourly with Serc (betahistidine hydrochloride) 16 mg six-hourly, inhalations of carbon dioxide 5% (1 l/min for one hour) six-hourly. Stellate ganglion blockade may also be used to promote inner ear circulation temporarily. Anoxic effects on intracellular metabolism may be alleviated by the use of steroids given for four days in therapeutic doses (Decadron (dexamethasone) 2 mg orally six-hourly) and then reduced the zero over a seven-day period. Hospital admission is essential so that the 'crash course of therapy', as indicated above, can be supervised with audiometric and electrolytic control and also so that the possibility of background vascular and endocrine disease can be thoroughly investigated.

Ménière's disease is a fairly clearly-defined and specific example of inner ear circulatory disorder in which an increase in endolymphatic volume (hydrops) is followed by distention of the membranous ducts of the labyrinth.

The patient suffers from recurrent attacks of acute vertigo accompanied by roaring tinnitus and sensory hearing loss. Acute vertigo for one to two hours is followed by degrees of imbalance and ataxia for one to two weeks. The attacks tends to come in clusters and with succeeding attacks, both the intensity of the tinnitus and its tendency to persist between attacks, and the degree of hearing loss, tend to increase. In uncontrolled Ménière's disease the hearing will often eventually deteriorate to a considerable degree.

In the acute phase, vertigo is the predominant symptom and is usually accompanied by nausea and vomiting. At the onset of an attack, horizontal nystagmus can be observed with the fast component towards the affected ear. Although the patient may not experience deafness or tinnitus initially, these will usually develop. Treatment consists of bed rest, sedation of the patient, and sedation of the vestibule. Valium (diazepam) in high doses is the drug of choice both for its tranquillizing effect and also its specific reregulating effect on the vestibular nuclei. Valium (diazepam) 10 mg, for an adult weighing 70 kg, should be given six-hourly.

If the patient is hospitalized, Valium (diazepam) is most effective if given intramuscularly, six-hourly. If the patient is at home, Valium (diazepam) can be commenced intramuscularly and continued orally for one to two weeks. Vasodilator therapy should be started as soon as possible and conists of maximum doses of Opilon (thymoxamine) 80 mg six-hourly and Serc (betahistidine hydrochloride) 16 mg six-hourly.

As soon as possible, the patient should be referred to an ENT clinic for complete otological and general medical assessment. Maintenance treatment with vasodilators and a labyrinthine sedative will then usually be continued for several months. Should the symptoms fail to be controlled in this way, one of several surgical treatments may be employed either to decompress the distended membranous labyrinth (which is the basic pathologic entity in Ménière's disease) if useful hearing still remains (Fig. 18), or alternatively, to eliminate the abnormal afferent input by total or selective destruction of the end-organ or its afferent neural pathways (labyrinthectomy or vestibular nerve section).

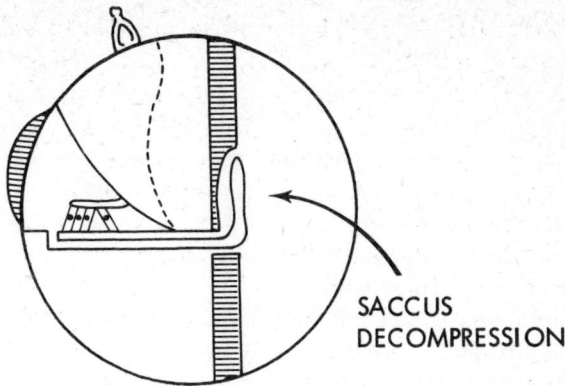

Fig. 18. Decompression of the endolymphatic space can be carried out by (a) puncturing the distended membranous duct when it has reached the deep surface of the stapes, through the stapes footplate; (b) creating a space in the bone around the saccus endolymphaticus.

A specific, not uncommon and probably inherited example of ischaemic failure is *strial atrophy*. In this, structural depletion of the 'power house' results in diminished electrical potential. The cochlea, being otherwise normal, now requires a stronger stimulus. Clinically, usually in middle life, the audiometric thresholds are bilaterally and uniformly elevated, but because speech discrimination remains good, amplification with two hearing aids (normal hearing is a bilateral function) is usually helpful.

(b) *Metabolic.* The cochlea is a highly dynamic organ. Anything which affects its energy supplies adversely will cause hearing loss — one such, ischaemia, has already been considered.

Another important factor in this category is thyroid dysfunction. The cochlea requires an adequate quantity of thyroxine and without this, as in even minor degrees of hypothyroidism, hearing diminishes.

As distinct from other types of sensory hearing loss, although the audiogram shows depression of function, this is characteristically bilateral, symmetrical, and affects all frequencies equally, giving a 'flat response' at about 40 dB through the speech frequencies. In addition, characteristic mucosal changes of hypothyroidism may be visible in the nose and larynx. On enquiry the patient will admit to 'feeling cold all the time; having to wear an extra sweater'. The diagnosis is based on biochemical tests.

Treatment with thyroxine will often produce a significant improvement in auditory function.

(c) *Ototoxicity*. A number of therapeutic agents have a specific damaging effect on the cochlea. These include aspirin, quinine, antibiotics such as streptomycin, gentamicin, kanamycin, and neomycin, diuretics such as Lasix (frusemide) and ethacrynic acid, and practically all antiseptic agents — if these are placed in the middle ear they can pass freely through the round window membrane into the cochlea with resultant destruction of hair cells. Cochlear damage from all of these substances, except aspirin, may be severe and can be prevented only by their absolute avoidance, especially if renal function is already poor, in all but life-threatening situations.

(d) *Presbycusis* — the hardness of hearing which comes to all of us, but in varied degree, with the passage of time.

This is basically a degenerative condition of the cochlea and its central connections and thus is a combined sensory and neural lesion.

The patient's age and degree of physical deterioration certainly suggest the diagnosis, but these should never prevent examination of the ear canals and TM to identify concomitant conductive problems due to wax, COM, or CSOM, and whose treatment in the former two instances will produce useful improvement in the patient's problem.

After the exclusion of any obvious conductive cause of hearing loss the diagnosis will be evident in most cases.

The age and rate at which presbycusis occurs is very variable. Hearing deteriorates in the senior citizen because of hair cell and neuronal loss due to vascular insufficiency, coupled with a loss of elasticity of the membranous inner ear. Under optimum conditions the effects of the process will not become apparent till the sixties at which time the patient will complain of hearing badly in noisy environments and request that enunciation should be clear but not over-loud (which causes distortion).

However, there are very few cochlea which reach middle age free from the effects of a series of aggressive influences since the earliest days of life. These include noise from road traffic, aircraft, industry, sport, discothèques, and military service. The effects of tobacco smoke, various therapeutic drugs, unremembered head injuries of varied degrees, circulatory impairment, metabolic dysfunction, childhood ASOM, and the possibility of an inherited deficiency of hair cells, all play their part. All of these can act singly or in combination to induce such a poverty of reserve that presbycusis often becomes apparent earlier than expected.

Treatment is certainly not curative but many patients are helped by reassurance that they are not in the process of going 'stone deaf' (which is very unusual in this group). Amplification of sound by means of a hearing aid is often helpful when used in quiet surroundings (but definitely not when there is background noise). However, some patients find the effect of a hearing aid disappointing, usually because of a greatly exaggerated disparity between the low-tone and high-tone responses — greater than that which is characteristically seen in the elderly patient's audiogram. This situation is not much assisted by simple amplification, and consonant reception, upon which word-identification largely depends, remains a problem. In spite of this, an appropriate hearing aid designed to give preferential high-tone boost should always be tried and the patient given sympathetic advice about his problem and the means of ameliorating it. In conjunction with a hearing aid, some tuition in lip-reading in those with functional vision can be helpful. Arrangements for hearing aid appraisal and lip-reading classes can best be made through the audiological department of the community hospital.

Lesions of the neural apparatus

These involve (i) the auditory nerve, (ii) the cochlear nuclei, and (iii) the second-order neuronal pathways which ascend through the brain stem to the auditory cortex in the temporal lobe.

The causes of such lesions can be categorized as congenital, traumatic, inflammatory, neoplastic, and 'others'.

Congenital causes

There is a variety of rare developmental defects which result in partial or total agenesis of the cochlea and the auditory nerve, either singly or in combination. Deafness is extreme and bilateral As is to be expected, audiological management can provide only limited assistance. Defects of other organ systems commonly co-exist and thus management of the auditory problems is only part of the overall care of these children.

Diagnosis is based on lack of speech development, a family history which is commonly present, developmental abnormalities of the pinna and meatus, and the findings on audiological assessment of gross perceptive hearing loss.

Treatment, as for other congenital losses, comprises amplification, tuition in lip-reading and speech therapy, usually on an institutionalized basis, coupled with the management of psychological and other medical problems.

Traumatic causes

Head injury not infrequently causes traction injury to the eighth nerve or concussive injury to the brain stem. This can occur at any age and is diagnosed from the history and the findings of perceptive hearing loss which is usually due to a combined sensory and neural defect.

Although *treatment* is rarely helpful, the possible value of amplification and lip-reading must be explored in every case.

Inflammatory causes

Viral infections (measles, chickenpox, herpes) of the brain stem and its neural connections, and bacterial and viral infections of the meninges are responsible for many of these neural hearing losses. Again the diagnosis is based on the history and a lack of other possible causes.

Amplification is rarely helpful owing to the gross lack of afferent pathway, but lip-reading has a part to play in the management of those patients with central dysfunction.

Neoplastic and other causes

(a) *Eighth nerve pathway lesions.* These are most often due to involvement of the auditory nerve by a tumour of the vestibular nerve (acoustic neurinoma). Tinnitus and hearing loss occur early in the disease, whereas imbalance is not often complained of because of gradual compensation at brain stem level. It should be noted that acoustic neurinoma frequently occurs in patients with Von Recklinghausen's disease.

The outcome for the patient depends upon early diagnosis and upon the awareness of all those who deal with patients suffering from hearing problems that *all unilateral perceptive hearing loss must be presumed to be caused by acoustic neurinoma until it can be proved otherwise.*

As a rule, the only positive findings on examination are (i) perceptive hearing loss, and (ii) imperfect performance of routine tests of balance.

The *diagnosis* is based on (i) a high index of suspicion, (ii) audiometry, (iii) tomographic studies of the internal auditory meatuses, and (iv) contrast studies of the posterior fossa and the internal auditory meatuses (this requires hospital admission). Note that all adult patients with unilateral perceptive hearing loss should be evaluated in depth so that the diagnosis of acoustic neurinoma can be confirmed or excluded as quickly as possible, hopefully while the tumour is still operative.

Other less common tumours arising in the internal auditory meatus present a similar clinical picture and these include congenital cholesteatoma, meningioma, and neuroma of the facial nerve.

(b) *Brain stem lesions*. These cause deafness because of involvement of the afferent pathways of the auditory nerve in the brain stem, the cochlear nuclei, and the immediate part of the second-order neurone.

Progressive hearing loss (especially affecting discrimination for speech) and imbalance are often combined with defects in oculomotor, seventh, ninth, and tenth nerve function. The differential diagnosis is between space-occupying lesions (tumours), vascular insufficiency, and demyelination of the neural pathways. With tumours there is an unrelenting progression of dysfunction whereas, by contrast, with ischaemic and sclerotic lesions, changes in symptoms and function tend to be much more fluctuant with a less precipitous course. Nevertheless, the general outlook is oppressive: only fair for vascular defects; extremely bad for demyelinating lesions; and hopeless for tumours (almost always glioma). No cause for deafness will be discovered through routine ENT examination and the diagnosis will eventually be achieved through neurological and radiological investigations.

Patients suffering from vascular insufficiency of the brain stem may be helped by general measures aimed at increasing oxygen perfusion such as through long-term therapy with Opilon (thymoxamine hydrochloride), Serc (bethahistine hydrochloride), or carbon dioxide inhalation.

The effects of multiple sclerotic plaques on brain stem function *may* be alleviated by the use of steroids, but supportive evidence for this claim is still lacking. Although tumours of the brain stem have been treated with temporary success by radiotherapy, the outcome is usually fatal.

HEARING AIDS

All hearing aids comprise a microphone, an amplifier, and a receiver. They are most often useful for conduction hearing loss but they also can be helpful in certain forms of sensorineural loss. Although the amount of assistance which any hard-of-hearing individual can expect from an aid can be predicted with fair accuracy by special tests of hearing, the most certain way of reaching a decision is by trying one or several aids in the environment where help is most needed. Although behind-the-ear or glasses-frame aids are often preferred (because they are less conspicuous and 'hear' at ear level), their performance is less satisfactory than the body aid in cases of extreme deafness. Unfortunately, none gives the high fidelity required for musical appreciation.

CONCLUSION

The causes of deafness are multiple and their diagnosis constitutes a considerable problem for all those who try to be of assistance to the unfortunate patient.

The prime role of the doctor working outside an otological clinic should be:

(1) to identify those patients whose problem is amenable to treatment;

(2) to treat the patient himself in the practice whenever possible and thus accelerate a successful outcome and also shorten hospital waiting lists;

(3) to allocate diagnosis and treatment to those specially trained in otology whenever the cause or treatment of the condition is obscure or out of the scope of community medicine.

5. Tinnitus

The transmission of environmental sounds to the auditory cortex depends upon:

(1) its amplification by the transformer mechanism of the middle ear, and

(2) the response to variations in the continuous flow of ions from the scala media to the scala tympani.

Tinnitus can occur:

(i) if the normal conduction mechanism, which gives preferential treatment to extraneous sound, including speech, is defective. Then endogenous sound may become audible both because the differential between it and speech is reduced, and also because less meaningful environmental sound no longer plays its part in obscuring body-generated sound (masking). Heartbeat tinnitus during catarrhal otitis media is a common example of this mechanism.

(ii) when the ion flow through the organ of Corti becomes changed or the response of the hair cells and neurones alters. This may lead to the generation of an abnormal signal, frequency-related to the affected part of the cochlea. A similar effect may result from faults in the efferent system of the cochlea (olivo-cochlear bundle) whose normal role is thought to be control of the level of transmitted electrical activity.

Presentation. Patients with tinnitus do not appear to be unwell unless there is an inflammatory or neoplastic cause or unless they have become psychologically disturbed by their symptoms. Their general state is determined by the disease which itself is responsible for their tinnitus. Because tinnitus can be a symptom of every and any form of auditory and aural disorder, questions should be specially designed to reveal the clues which will lead to discovering the cause. For example, the possibility of noise exposure, certain medications, and endocrine and metabolic disease should always be considered. Very obviously the diagnosis of tinnitus can pose a formidable challenge in terms of problem-solving.

The difficulties are less if we are aware of the almost universal association of tinnitus with hearing defects. If it is presumed that both symptoms when they occur together have the same cause, then the evaluation of tinnitus, which would be impossible *per se* because of its entirely subjective nature, can be carried out indirectly through tests of auditory function. Therefore the investigation of tinnitus is essentially the same as the investigation of deafness. Consequently, in practice, we can classify tinnitus as being due to lesions of:

(1) the *external ear canal,* such as impacted wax and the debris of chronic external otitis;

(2) *the middle ear,* such as in acute and catarrhal otitis media and otosclerosis;

(3) *the inner ear* including virtually all the causes of sensory hearing loss, the degenerative and traumatic being the most common; and

(4) *the afferent pathways,* of which the most important lesions are acoustic neurinoma and brain stem ischaemia.

Patients describe their symptom by comparing it with normal environmental sounds such as the hum of wind in telephone wires, the roar of waves beating on the coast, the noise of a combustion engine, the hiss of escaping steam, the whistle which emanates from television sets at the close of transmission, or the pounding of their heartbeat.

High-pitched tinnitus is characteristic of lesions caused by exposure to high-intensity noise (in industry and from gunfire and bomb blast) and in presbycusis, whereas low-frequency roaring and 'engine noise' is typical of Ménière's disease.

Although most tinnitus is continuous, it can be intermittent and of variable intensity as in Ménière's disease, or temporary as in finite middle ear disorders. Its effect varies largely because of differences in the underlying disorder but partly because of the individual's reaction to it. The patient's response is not always constant and tolerance is often diminished by stress, worry, and other diseases.

Treatment. The frequently heard advice: 'So you've got a noise in your head. We can do nothing about it—go away and learn to live with it' is both inhumane and also not necessarily always factually correct.

The patient deserves a full, honest, and sympathetic explanation of the nature of his disorder so that his natural anxiety about underlying sinister disease or a worsening of the symptom in the future does not exaggerate the severity of his symptom.

Disorders of middle ear function can often be corrected by stapedectomy or tympanoplasty, with improvement or even cure of tinnitus. Eliminating aspirin from the regime of the arthritic patient rapidly stops tinnitus and when the administration of amino-glycoside antibiotics is complicated by tinnitus this can be limited or terminated by changing the drug. The correction of metabolic disorders such as diabetes or hypothyroidism is often dramatic in its effect on tinnitus. The elimination of anaemia and the control of hypertension, hypercholesterolaemia, and other circulatory diseases can offer much to the patient whose presenting symptom is 'head-noises'.

When ischaemic inner ear disease is accelerating the progressive degenerative disorders associated with ageing, vasodilators such as thymoxamine are sometimes effective in halting or retarding the process. When noises exposure is inevitable, then advice about ear protection can prevent worsening of tinnitus.

Finally, advice about ways of providing background noise to reduce the patient's awareness of tinnitus (quietly played radio music, a loudly ticking clock) and therapeutically induced suppression with tranquillizers and sleeping tablets may play an important part in the management of this disturbing complaint. Fortunately, for the majority of patients the symptom, or their reaction to it, tends to become less with time.

REVISION: THE CAUSES OF DEAFNESS AND TINNITUS

For revision purposes, the causes of deafness and tinnitus can be listed as follows:

1. **Conductive** due to:
   - (a) obstruction of the external auditory meatus
     - (i) wax
     - (ii) foreign bodies
     - (iii) swellings
   - (b) diseases of the sound-transforming mechanism
     - (i) acute suppurative otitis media
     - (ii) chronic catarrhal otitis media
     - (iii) chronic suppurative otitis media
     - (iv) otosclerosis
     - (v) carcinoma of the middle ear

2. **Perceptive or sensorineural** due to lesions of the
   (a) stria vascularis
       (i) congenital atrophy
       (ii) salicylate intoxication
       (iii) vascular occlusion
   (b) inner ear fluids
       (i) Ménière's disease
       (ii) syphilitic labyrinthitis
       (iii) vascular occlusion
   (c) organ of Corti
       (i) congenital absence
       (ii) trauma
           (1) noise and blast
           (2) fracture
       (iii) ototoxicity
       (iv) labyrinthitis
   (d) basilar membrane
       (i) degenerative — presbycusis
   (e) nerve cells and fibres of auditory nerve
       (i) degenerative — presbycusis
       (ii) acoustic neurinoma
       (iii) multiple sclerosis
       (iv) fracture of the petrous bone
       (v) vascular occlusion

6. Dizziness

The first attack of dizziness is a terrifying experience, frequently thought by the patient, and often his doctor, to indicate a brain tumour or cerebrovascular accident. Although disorders of balance can be due to central nervous disease, the majority have an otological cause and require investigation and treatment in an ENT department.

The function of the balancing mechanism can be linked to that of a computer system. Obviously, disorders of any part of the computer will effect its efficiency. Therefore, we would expect that dizziness could be due to disease of the labyrinth, the brain stem, or of the efferent system. In fact, the most common causes of dizziness are those which affect the labyrinth, with brain stem disease accounting for most of the remainder. When the relationship which normally exists between the output of each labyrinth is disturbed because of a disproportionate alteration in the electrical activity of *one* labyrinth, such as occurs during the stimulation of a caloric test or because of unilateral depression due to temporal bone fracture or labyrinthine infection, then the brain stem will receive information, which in the light of its past learned responses, it cannot interpret, and therefore it inevitably distributes false information to the rest of the body.

A similar situation will arise when correct information from the labyrinth is misinterpreted by a diseased brain stem. Because information reaching the cortex does not correlate with data from other sources, there is confusion, i.e. an hallucination of movement, or vertigo. The eyes repeatedly seek the last field of gaze, so we have nystagmus. Peristalsis ceases and may even be reversed, so there is nausea and even vomiting. The muscles are prepared for a state of affairs which never actually occurs, and consequently, we have ataxia. This 'crisis' situation is characteristic of that which always occurs when either (i) the balance of correct and proportionate electrical activities of the two labyrinths is disturbed, or (ii) the analytical processes of the brain stem are disordered.

The clinical problem

In the **labyrinth,** three distinct types of crisis situation can occur (Fig. 19):

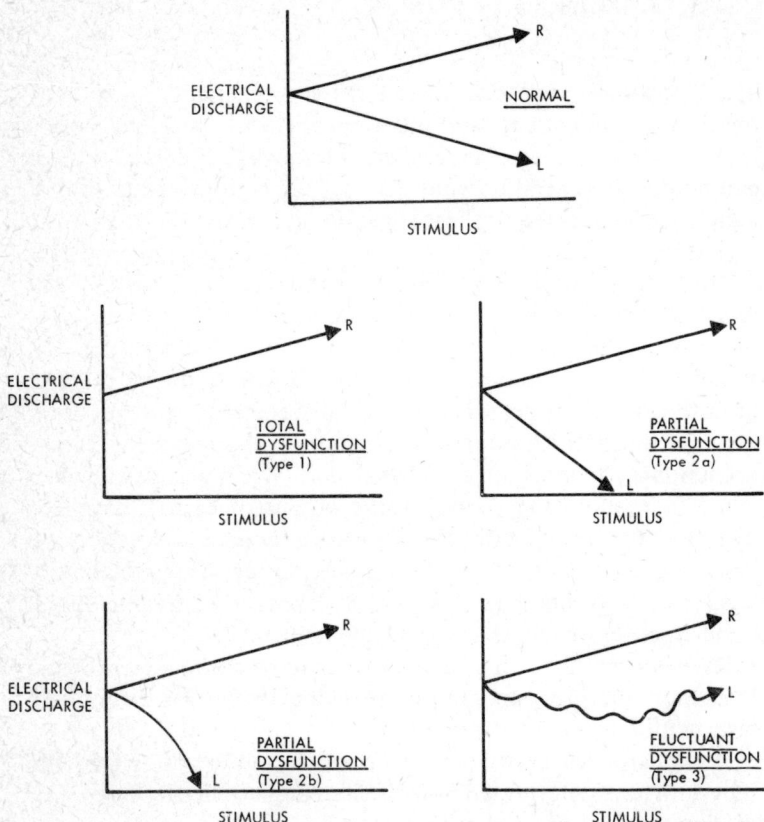

Fig. 19. Under normal circumstances (L = left, R = right) the stimulus due to a positional chance from rest produces a labyrinthine response which is linear and in which the electrical activity of one labyrinth changes at an equal rate to the other, but has an opposite value so that the *total* output is unchanged. In unilateral labyrinthine disease the ipsilateral electrical discharge varies and is related to the type and extent of the lesion.

1. **Total unilateral cessation of function** due to fracture of the petrous bone, surgical trauma to the labyrinth, total occlusion of the inner ear vasculature, viral infection of the vestibular nerves and Scarpa's ganglion (vestibular neuronitis), drug intoxication

(e.g. with streptomycin and the other aminoglycoside antibiotics), and round window membrane rupture due to abrupt changes in atmospheric pressure.

2. **Partial dysfunction** due to less extensive vascular accidents and virus disease causing postural and positional vertigo.

3. **Fluctuant alterations in function** caused by (a) hydropic metabolic disorders of the inner ear, such as in Ménière's disease and its variants, and (b) intermittent fistulae of the round and oval windows.

In the **brain stem** two types of crisis situation arise:

1. **Total or partial cessation of function** because of tumour or vascular occlusion.

2. **Fluctuant alterations in function** due to demyelinating or transitory vascular disease.

LABYRINTHINE DISEASE

Type 1

The brain stem response which follows unilateral labyrinthine destruction provides a blueprint upon which attempts to treat lesser forms of disease can be designed. It is now known that following the experimental termination of afferent information from one labyrinth, an inhibitive effect from the cerebellum completely suppresses the ipsilateral medial vestibular nucleus and reduces by half the activity of the contralateral nucleus. This modifying effect lasts for between one and two weeks during which, although acute vertigo is experienced, its degree is doubtless much less than would be the case without central suppression. Gradually, electrical activity in the ipsilateral nucleus begins to return until eventually it matches that of the contralateral nucleus, which simultaneously and gradually returns to normal. During this recovery period, the brain stem starts to resume its co-ordinate processes but now on the basis of the input from only one labyrinth instead of two, and eventually through a process of re-education, many patients find that they are reasonably free from incapacitating vestibular symptoms. Obviously the chances of such an outcome are directly related to the health of the brain stem.

Type 2

When labyrinthine destruction is less than total, although vertigo may be initially as acute as in the Type 1 situation, the eventual outcome will depend upon the degree of permanent damage. Type 2 labyrinthine dysfunction can be separated clinically into two groups:

2(a) When damage is relatively minor, then the brain stem may learn to interpret a new signal which, though admittedly not normal, is *constant,* and eventually *predictable,* and quite soon, changes of posture can be performed reasonably well.

2(b) When there is extensive damage, because of excessive fatiguability and other factors inherent in neuronal degeneration, the response to larger stimuli may be less satisfactory. Although fortunately the overall problem can be helped in many instances by medication and physiotherapy, nevertheless, the afferent input from a badly affected labyrinth may continue to be so out of phase with that of its fellow that a meaningful response pattern can never be re-established. In this situation (Type 2(b)), surgical treatment can be helpful if it eliminates this disruptive input and creates for the brain stem a situation which pertains in Type 1 situation.

The accompanying vertigo

Two specific and separate entities are recognized clinically:

(i) **Postural change vertigo** in which (1) sudden alterations in total body posture as occurs, for example, on suddenly arising from bed, or (2) rapid changes in cervical musculo-skeletal input, such as occur in reaching to a high shelf, are followed by loss of balance. Postural change vertigo is the residuum of an acute labyrinthine disorder of Type 1 or Type 2 category and occurs either because of an inadequate response to a large stimulus or because of a temporary breakdown in brain stem compensation due to a febrile illness, excessive tiredness, or stress. Similar symptoms also occur in patients suffering from cervical arthritis or following whiplash injury in whom a sudden (unexpected) abnormal afferent input disturbs the proper workings of the 'computer analyser'.

(ii) **Positional vertigo,** often described as paroxysmal and benign, occurs on the assumption of specific positions, usually in bed. Characteristically, some seconds after turning to one side, the patient experiences acute vertigo. The diagnosis of this condition is confirmed by the observation of rotatory nystagmus when the patient is placed in the critical position. This is thought to be the end-result of occlusion of the utricular artery followed by the release of calcium particles from the degenerating macula. These flow into the posterior semicircular canal and stimulate its crista when the head is in the appropriate position.

Type 3

Hydrops can affect all or part of the labyrinth. Thus, its clinical presentation varies from acute vertigo alone to acute vertigo with hearing loss, tinnitus, and 'pressure' in the ear. When all of these are combined the condition is called Ménière's disease but many patients suffer from one or other symptom independently.

Background

A brief review of current attitudes of labyrinthine hydrops is necessary to explain our therapeutic approach to these patients.

The inner ear is a complicated two-compartment system of fluids, perilymph and endolymph, which differ in ionic composition. Perilymph originates both from cerebrospinal fluid passing from the cochlear aqueduct to the scala vestibuli and from vessels in the lining of the scala vestibuli, whence it passes around the helicotrema to the scala tympani. During its passage along this course, perilymph passes through Reissner's membrane into the scala media and is converted into endolymph by the action of the stria vascularis (a metabolic power house) so that it becomes rich in potassium and low in sodium content. Some endolymph is probably absorbed by the lining membrane of the scala media and some may cross back through Reissner's membrane but most passes longitudinally along the ductus endolymphaticus where it is absorbed in the saccus endolymphaticus. It is believed that failure of endolymph absorption by the saccus endolymphaticus is the primary cause of the over-accumulation of fluid in the scala media (hydrops) which subsequently leads to distention and distortion of the inner ear membranes, impairment of their function, and eventually even structural defects leading to mixing of the fluids which results in hair cell destruction and finally neuronal death. Thus, hydrops arises from malabsorption of endolymph, and progresses to permanent distortion of the inner ear membranes and loss of their function. It appears likely that the initial problem is vascular — a microcirculatory failure of the absorptive mechanisms of the saccus endolymphaticus (Fig. 17).

The disease

In the *early stages* of hydrops, i.e. for as long as the basis of the problem remains vasospastic and presumably reversible, the electrical activity of the affected labyrinth is characteristically fluctuant, and constantly unpredictable — not a good basis for the re-establishment of a workable analyser: its output is not only constantly, but also irregularly, out of phase with that of its partner. If vasospasm proceeds to thrombosis, then the stage of potential reversibility is over: fluctuations in electrical activity will cease and there will now be a Type 2 situation in which the input will be constant and possibly eventually predictable. Clearly, both situations pose considerable interpretative problems at brain stem level and many patients find it difficult or even impossible to retrain their brain stem coding systems in order to regain equilibrium.

If any form of *treatment,* medical or surgical, can affect hydrops successfully in its early stages, then it will do so by normalizing endolymphatic metabolism. When the fluctuant and potentially reversible phase of the disease has passed, then surgical treatment can be effective only if it frees the brain stem analyser from the input of a permanently and largely disordered end-organ.

Treatment

The last section attempted to explain why a proportion of patients in Types 2 and 3 cannot be helped by medical means. Fortunately for many of these tragic cases, modern developments in the surgical treatment of inner ear diseases have led to a considerable improvement in their prospects of rehabilitation.

BRAIN STEM DISEASE

Type 1

Gross damage to the vestibular nuclei results in acute ataxia due to impairment of the central analysis of afferent input which is reflected in a disordered efferent output. When this is due to a tumour or a thrombotic vascular lesion the effect is likely to be permanent and frequently associated with other cranial nerve defects.

Type 2

Temporary or partial recovery from the effects of demyelinating disease or lesser vascular disturbances (short of infarction) is usual.

Vertigo with acute onset will subside within days or weeks, in parallel with the restoration of brain stem function. There may also be associated deafness because of concomitant auditory nerve involvement.

INVESTIGATION OF THE DIZZY PATIENT

Preliminary

First, obtain a history of the character, frequency, and duration of the attacks of imbalance; enquire about recent infections, head trauma, drugs, and general health, with questions specific to disorders of metabolism and circulation; and examine fully the nose and throat, and especially the ears. Secondly evaluate the patient's ability to defend his equilibrium. This is done quite simply by observing the patient's posture at rest, while standing with eyes open and closed, on both feet together and on one foot, and his ability to walk with eyes open and closed.

Audiometric studies

In the investigation of the dizzy patient audiometric studies are essential. Pure tone threshold and speech tests evaluate the auditory mechanisms in general terms. These are augmented by special tests, which include tone decay and loudness balance tests, of the neural pathways between the end-organ and the brain stem. In special situations, complex tests of the mid-brain's ability to code and dicotomize information are used. Again the site of the lesion may be designated to the temporal lobe by EEG tests of cortical function augmented by EMI scanning.

Caloric and positional testing

The vestibular mechanisms are evaluated by means of positional and caloric testing. In the caloric test, the response of the labyrinth to stimulation by temperature change are compared. Electronystagmographic records of the eye movements (ENG) are used to make a permanent record of the results of these tests and provide a number of parameters, including frequency, eye speed, waveform, and duration, which can be recorded and measured.

Positional tests evaluate both the function of the utricle and the neck reflexes and the results are also recorded by ENG. In all of these tests, the nystagmoid beat is enhanced by having the patient's eyes closed and by using mental distraction techniques in the form of counting backwards in twos from 100. Because of the close relationship of other cranial nerves with the eighth cranial nerve, the motor and sensory function of the third to tenth cranial nerves should always be evaluated.

Other investigations

In addition, the blood pressure, carotid pulses, and neck mobility should be noted routinely. Blood tests should include the FTA-abs. test, peripheral blood films, blood cholesterol, and T_3 and T_4 levels. Chest and skull X-rays and tomographic films of the internal auditory meatus are routinely performed to detect metastatic and primary neoplastic causes of vertigo.

TREATMENT

Initially, in any **acute** disorder of balance the first aim of treatment is to sedate the patient and sedate the vestibular mechanisms. Valium (diazepam) is one of the most suitable drugs for both purposes and should be given in maximum doses. If the patient can be admitted to hospital, diazepam is given intramuscularly in doses up to 25 mg in 24 hours. When the basic aetiology is thought to be vascular, either primarily, or as a consequence of virus infection, any means of promoting the microcirculation of the inner ear and its central connections should be considered. These include carbon dioxide inhalations (5 l/min of 5% CO_2 with 95% O_2 for one hour three times daily), Opilon (thymoxamine) 80 mg three times daily, Serc (betahistine hydrochloride) 16 mg three times daily, nicotinic acid 100 mg three times daily, and stellate ganglion blockage.

Labyrinthine lesions

In labyrinthine lesions, when there is permanent and total loss of peripheral function (**Type 1**), recovery will occur spontaneously as the result of the establishment of a new brain stem mechanism. Treatment is aimed at supporting the patient through this period.

In **Type 2** patients, when the end-organ defect is partial, a new but predictable pattern of afferent activity will often be established and function well in response to moderate stimuli. This process can be assisted by vestibular sedation with drugs such as Stemetil (prochlorperazine maleate) 5 mg three times daily, Dramamine (dimenhydrinate) 25 mg three times daily, or Stugeron (cinnarizine) 15 mg daily. Progress towards recovery can frequently be associated by physiotherapy (Cooksey's exercises).

However, when the defect is greater and the afferent input is so out of phase with that of the other labyrinth that a meaningful response can never be re-established then 'medical' therapy is usually ineffective. In such circumstances, surgical treatment aimed at ridding the brain stem from the distracting influence of the disordered labyrinth either by labyrinthectomy or vestibular nerve section creates the situation of the patient in Type 1 in which the brain stem can re-establish a new programme based on the input from one single normal labyrinth.

In **Type 3** patients, where hydrops of the labyrinth is responsible for vertigo, treatment is aimed in the early stages at promoting the microcirculation of the inner ear, as outlined earlier. These therapies will often be effective if commenced *early* in the course of the disease. However, when vertigo becomes incapacitating in Ménière's disease and cannot be controlled by medications the only possible solution is a surgical one.

If useful hearing is still present in the affected ear (and this is the rule even in advanced Ménière's disease) then an operation which preserves residual cochlear function (either vestibular nerve section or decompression of the saccus endolymphaticus) is indicated. The importance of preserving hearing cannot be overestimated in a disease which will eventually affect the second ear in 25 per cent of patients. However, when all auditory function has ceased in the affected ear, usually from causes other than Ménière's disease, then the patient can best be assisted by disassociation from his abnormal vestibular afferent input by total labyrinthectomy, in which all of the inner ear structures are destroyed surgically.

Brain stem lesions

Treatment is aimed at supporting the patient by medications which will sedate the disordered vestibular mechanisms. As with peripheral lesions, Valium (diazepam), Stugeron (cinnarizine), and Stemetil (prochlorperazine maleate) are often helpful. When imbalance is caused by a tumour, palliation is all that can be hoped for; when a vascular or demyelinating lesion is present, although recovery may be attributed to therapy, it should be rocognized that this may well be the result of a spontaneous remission.

There is a small group of patients whose symptoms arise neither peripherally nor centrally but from a tumour of the sheath of the vestibular nerve as it lies in the internal auditory meatus — an acoustic neurinoma, congenital cholesteatoma, or meningioma. In these patients the main complaint is of tinnitus and deafness. Although they may be ataxic when examined, these patients complain less about disorders of balance than they do about deafness and tinnitus. The confirmation or exclusion of an internal auditory meatus tumour can be made with certainty only on the basis of tomography of the internal auditory meatus, contrast studies of the posterior fossae, and the presence of increased levels of protein in the cerebrospinal fluid. Because these tumours eventually become inoperable due to involvement with the brain stem, an early diagnosis is highly desirable. **Early diagnosis is based on a high index of suspicion in all patients who have a unilateral perceptive hearing loss.** All such patients must be investigated until the possibility of a space-occupying lesion of the internal auditory meatus can be ruled out with certainty.

REVISION: CAUSES OF DIZZINESS

For revision purposes, the causes of imbalance can be listed as follows:

1. **Traumatic:**
    (a) changes in barometric pressure
    (b) concussion to labyrinth and eighth nerve
    (c) surgical — stapedectomy and tympanoplasty
    (d) fracture of petrous temporal bone

2. **Inflammatory:**
    labyrinthitis
    (a) viral
    (b) bacterial

3. **Neoplastic:**
    (a) carcinoma of middle ear
    (b) meningioma
    (c) acoustic neurinoma
    (d) congenital cholesteatoma
    (e) eosinophilic granuloma of the petrous bone

4. **Others:**
    (a) metabolic
        (i) hypothyroidism
        (ii) diabetes mellitus
        (iii) hormonal disturbance

(b) vascular
    (i) Ménière's disease
    (ii) brain stem lesions
(c) vascular/viral
    (i) neuronitis
        (1) labyrinth
        (2) eighth nerve
        (3) brain stem
(d) postural
    (i) neck
        (1) abnormal afferent input
        (2) vertebral arterial occlusion
    (ii) Type 2 lesion (limited response)
    (iii) loss central compensation
(e) benign paroxysmal
    (i) vascular defect
(f) drug-induced

7. Facial paralysis

Presentation

In upper motor neurone lesions due usually to cerebrovascular accident, frontalis movement is spared. In lower motor neurone lesions all divisions of the nerve may be affected. The rate of onset may be gradual or rapid, depending on the cause.

Causes

In identifying the reason for facial paralysis it is useful to separate traumatic, inflammatory, and neoplastic causes.

Traumatic causes of facial paralysis

There will be a clear history of either recent head injury or surgical treatment of the ear or parotid gland. The site of injury within the skull can be determined by X-ray and from the result of Schirmer's tearing test which is negative when the lesion is proximal to the greater superficial petrosal nerve and the geniculate ganglion.

Inflammatory causes of facial paralysis

These are:

1. *Middle ear infections* usually complicating cholesteatoma. The patient will usually give a history of prolonged otorrhoea and hearing loss. The TM and hearing levels should be examined thoroughly in every patient with facial weakness to exclude inflammatory causes.

2. Infections with *neutrotrophic viruses* are now thought to be responsible for a large number of the so-called idiopathic facial palsies (Bell's palsy). Other nerves may be involved also giving rise to dysfunction and a painful vesicular eruption (Ramsay Hunt syndrome).

The onset of Bell's palsy may be preceded or accompanied by severe pain around the ear. Its onset is usually sudden and often follows exposure to cold air. Paralysis is rarely immediately total but may advance rapidly and become total. Fortunately, at least three out of every four patients eventually recover spontaneously.

Neoplastic causes of facial paralysis

In contract to traumatic and inflammatory causes, the onset of facial weakness due to tumour involvement is usually very gradual but will become complete if the cause remains untreated.

A neuroma can occur in any part of the nerve's course but does so most commonly in the middle ear where it may also affect hearing and be visible through the tympanic membrane. Meningioma of the internal auditory meatus or the posterior fossa is an infrequent but occasional source of facial palsy, whereas acoustic neurinoma rarely affects the facial nerve's function.

Carcinoma of the middle ear is often not diagnosed until facial weakness gives warning of the sinister cause for signs and symptoms which so often masquerade as CSOM.

When facial paralysis occurs in association with a parotid swelling this is always because of the malignant nature of the tumour.

The diagnosis is based on the speed on onset, the health and function of the ear, the presence or absence of lacrymation, and the results of histological and radiological investigations.

Treatment

Facial paralysis due to trauma: It is important to establish whether facial paralysis was present from the time of injury or developed later. When there is a delay in onset, expectant treatment with steroids will be commenced at once, whereas if there was no delay, severe injury is presumed and surgical exploration, decompression, and grafting carried out as necessary.

In skull fracture, 90% of lesions are just lateral to the outer end of the internal auditory meatus. In order to expose the nerve in this area a combined otological–neurosurgical operation is performed using the middle fossa route.

Bell's palsy: A decade-old controversy over the relative merits of steroid and ACTH therapy as compared with surgical decompression is not yet resolved. In most centres, although treatment is primarily medical, the vitality of the nerve is monitored by electrical tests so that should there be signs of imminent neuronal degeneration, attempts can be made to increase the blood circulation of the nerve by opening the fallopian canal and slitting the nerve sheath (decompression operation).

Facial paralysis due to cholesteatomatous middle ear disease is treated by surgical means, supported by broad-spectrum antibiotic.

Tympanoplasty with maintenance of the ear canal wall is usually preferred to radical mastoidectomy because of the better healing and functional results obtained.

Decompression of the facial nerve for several millimeters in each direction away from the affected part of the nerve is usually performed to promote perineural blood flow.

Facial paralysis due to tumours. The site of involvement is identified on the basis of the results of auditory and vestibular tests, X-rays, and Schirmer's test. Treatment is by surgical means using the transmastoid, middle, or posterior fossa routes as is appropriate. When a tumour in the outer or middle ear is malignant, surgical treatment is usually combined with radiotherapy.

REVISION: THE CAUSES OF FACIAL PARALYSIS

For revision purposes, the causes of facial paralysis can be listed as follows:

1. **Upper motor neurone lesions,** due to
    (a) cerebrovascular accidents
    (b) penetrating brain injury
    (c) neoplasia

2. **Lower motor neurone lesions,** due to
    (a) temporal bone fracture
    (b) meningioma
    (c) acoustic neurinoma
    (d) facial nerve neuroma
    (e) cholesteatoma
    (f) acute suppurative otitis media
    (g) surgical trauma during middle ear and parotid gland operations
    (h) viral infections, e.g. Ramsay Hunt syndrome

The nose

8. Anatomy and physiology

The nasal cavity occupies the central position of the middle third of the face and extends from the nostrils to the posterior choanae where it joins with the nasopharynx. Communicating air spaces extend laterally into the maxilla (the antrum) and the ethmoid, superiorly into the frontal bone, and posteriorly into the sphenoid bone to form the accessory nasal sinuses (Fig. 20). The pyramidal

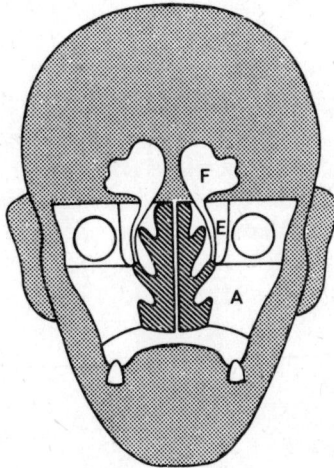

Fig. 20. The relationships of the accessory nasal sinuses. The ethmoidal sinuses (E) and maxillary antrum (A) lie medial and inferior to the orbit. The frontal sinus (F) develops from the anterior ethmoidal area.

shaped nasal cavity is bisected from front to back by the nasal septum and from each lateral wall three turbinates project into its lumen. The nasal cavity and its sinuses are lined by a ciliated mucous membrane which provides a transport system to maintain the health and function of the nose. A mucus blanket supported on the tips of cilia and in continuous movement posteriorly protects the lining membrane from pathogenic organisms, airborne irritants, and changes in the humidity and temperature of the inspired air (Fig. 21).

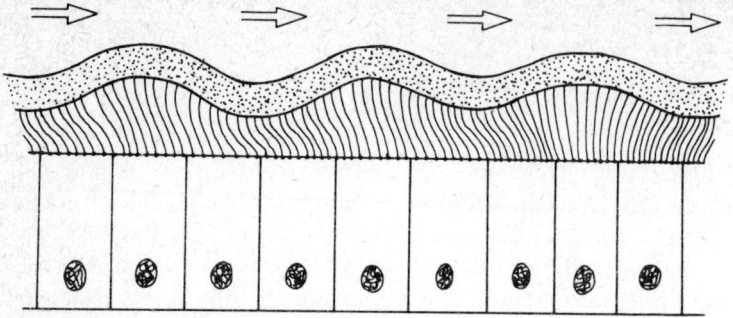

Fig. 21. The mucus blanket moves over the tips of cilia and acts as a conveyor belt which can move debris from the nostril to the posterior choana in 15 minutes.

The **function** of the nasal cavity is twofold:

1. To warm, moisten, and clean the air in preparation for alveolar exchange. In this, the inferior turbinate with its labile vascular supply and plentiful mucus glands plays an important part.

2. Olfaction. The roof of the nasal cavity is lined with a specialized neuroepithelium and mediates a chemical reaction with olfactory particles which results in an afferent input via the first cranial nerve to the olfactory cortex.

9. Nasal catarrh

'Catarrh' is commonplace in temperate climates. Many of those who complain about stuffy noses are also troubled by 'postnasal drip'. Although endocrine disorders and certain drugs may be responsible, the principal causes of these symptoms are:

(1) allergy,
(2) infection, and
(3) anatomic abnormalities

Frequently these act together.

ALLERGIC RHINITIS

Nasal allergy is the result of an altered reaction to foreign substances in the inspired air (Fig. 22) and can be classified as:

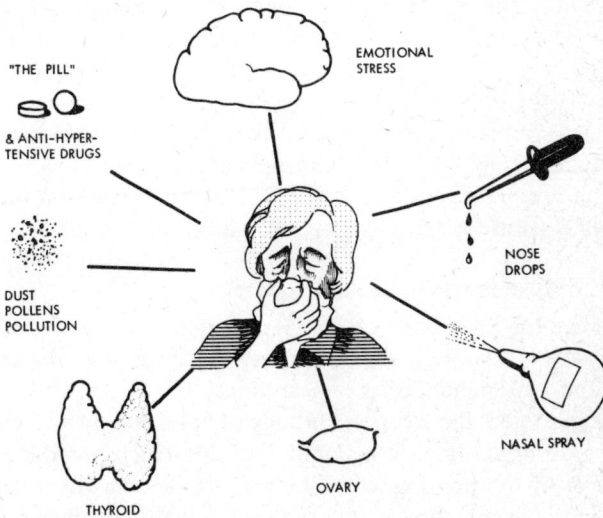

ALLERGIC AND NON-ALLERGIC CAUSES OF
OEDEMA OF THE NASAL AND SINUS MUCOSA

Fig. 22. Many different factors can provoke a vasomotor reaction in the nasal mucosa. Protein materials are often responsible for an allergic response leading to the release of histamine.

(1) **seasonal** ('hay fever'), in which the symptoms are due to pollens from trees and grasses to which exposure occurs only at certain times of the year; or

(2) **perennial,** in which the symptoms are caused by substances, such as house dust and animal dander, constantly present in the environment.

Mechanism of allergic reactions

The antigenic substances are usually proteins or combinations of non-protein and body protein (haptens). The antigen reacts abnormally with antibody within or on the surface of cells, releasing histamine. The pharmacological effects of this histamine are responsible for the symptoms of allergic rhinitis.

The basic mechanism of allergic reactions is the induction, in a predisposed cell, of a specific substance which is toxic in its action, by an antigen. The toxic substance then conjugates with the antigenic molecules to form an antibody which may be activated by another molecule of the same antigen when it subsequently enters the cell. This touches off a biochemical explosion of toxic proteolysis within the sensitized cell with the liberation of various toxins. At the end of this, the original antibody regenerates itself to be ready for another biochemical explosion, if more of the specific antigen should re-enter the sensitized cell. Thus, a self-perpetuating pathogenic mechanism is established within the cell, and this constitutes the primary mechanism of allergic reactions.

Actions of histamine in the nasal cavity

It is known that histamine causes (i) contraction of smooth muscle, (ii) capillary dilatation and increased permeability of capillary walls, and (iii) glandular hypersecretion.

We can predict the symptomatology of nasal allergy by considering the potential effect of histamine on the structures which form the lining of the nasal cavity. The vascular system consists of an arteriole which supplies a capillary network in the submucosa. Most of the blood in the capillary area flows from the arterial to the venous side through the metarteriole which acts as a bypass and feeds the capillary bed only when humoral effects (e.g. by histamine) cause relaxation of the precapillary sphincter. Normally, this control is autonomous and depends upon local metabolic requirements. The effect of histamine release is to produce statis of the nasal circulation. This is because relaxation of the muscle sphincter at the proximal end of the capillary results in flooding of the capillary bed, now secondarily dilated by histamine, with slowing of circulation and consequent hypoxia (and cyanosis) leading to accumulation of oedema fluid. These changes will occur especially in areas where the blood supply is well-developed, and in particular the mucosa of the inferior turbinate.

Simultaneously, histamine stimulation of the glandular structures will result in an over-production of mucus. Therefore on examining the allergic nose we would expect to find a pale, often cyanotic, swelling of the inferior turbinates, accompanied by an excessive amount of mucus secretion. **Inflammatory complications** may arise out of interference with the defence mechanism of the nasal mucosa which consists of the protective mucus blanket which protects the mucosal layer from inspired irritants and infectious agents, and regulates the exchange of fluid and heat between the nasal mucosa and the intranasal air. The success of this mucus blanket as a protective mechanism is based on its continuous renewel by secretion from the mucus glands of the lining membrane, coupled with its propulsion by the cilia of the columnar epithelium from the front to the back of the nose. Thus the mucus blanket is a **conveyor belt** which carries foreign material to the nasopharynx for disposal by swallowing into the acid content of the stomach. Although infectious elements trapped in the mucus blanket will be opposed by lysozymes and other substances with antiviral and antibacterial properties, it is important that these organisms be kept on the move to prevent the establishment of colonies with invasive qualities.

The mucus blanket is kept in continuous motion, not only by means of the cilia, but also by the milking effect of inspired air — each inspiration is a 'mini-sniff'. For this process to function the nasal mucus must be of the correct consistency, and volume. Any alteration in the character of the mucus secretion, or in the vitality of the columnar epithelium which arises from histamine release in the submucosa, will predispose to infectious complications.

Symptoms

Nasal obstruction is caused by mucosal swelling and the excessive production of tenacious mucus. **Sneezing** and **nasal discharge,** often in the form of 'postnasal drip', are frequently also present. Patients with allergic rhinitis often complain of **anosmia,** obstruction of the olfactory region of the nose, discomfort and **dryness of the throat, and cough,** due to the fact that in the absence of air-filtering, they are breathing cold, dry, and contaminated air directly through the mouth and into the throat. The patient sums up the situation with the statement that he **'always has a cold'.** If, because of impairment of the normal defence mechanisms, complications arise, then there may also be the signs and symptoms of sinusitis or otitis media.

Diagnosis

The diagnosis of nasal allergy is **usually obvious** from the history and clinical findings, and is confirmed by eosinophil counts of nasal secretion and the results of therapeutic trials with antihistamines, vaccines, and sometimes topical steroids.

The history

It is important to enquire from the patient himself about factors which he considers might be causative and also to find out as much as possible about potential causes in the patient's environment at home and in his work. Many patients in industry are in contact with allergens; at home, house dust, the dander of animals or birds, and pollens from the garden may be identified. A family history of allergy is an important clue and it may well be that the patient has relatives with other manifestations of allergy, such as asthma or dermatitis.

Clinical examination

Preliminary conversation with the patient makes it apparent that there is an impairment of vocal resonance (rhinolalia clausa) due to a lack of patency of the intranasal space. When the nasal tip is tilted upwards by the examiner's thumb the nasal mucosa can be examined by torch light. Its appearance is usually diagnostic — the inferior turbinates are enlarged, pale, boggy, and often lilac-coloured. Sticky secretions form strands between the septum and the turbinates. The overall swelling and pallor of the nasal mucosa is impressive. These appearances are explained by the histological appearances of biopsy tissue, in which the mucosal layer is many cells thicker than normal, with enlarged rete pegs. The cells and fibres of the submucosal layer are widely separated by oedematous fluid which is infiltrated by eosinophils. In adult cases of perennial allergy, nasal obstruction is often aggravated by the presence of polypi. These are pale, grape-like swellings which project from the middle and superior meatuses into the nasal lumen. With time these become larger, and eventually cause total obstruction of nasal breathing. Usually polyps can be clearly seen through the nostrils with torch illumination but should not be confused with an *allergically enlarged inferior turbinate* which lies laterally in the *inferior third* of the intranasal space.

Polyps arise from the ethmoidal cells, and are the product of mucosal oedema which, as it proceeds and the lumen of the cells becomes obliterated, results in protrusion of the swollen mucosa through the ostium of the cell into the nasal airway. Continued exposure to allergens leads to a further enlargements of this protrusion into a polyp, and this is added to by the traction effect of nose-blowing and forcible breathing. Narrowness of the sinus ostium impedes venous return and this increases the oedema of the projecting mucosa with enlargement of the polyp (Fig. 23). On X-ray, the appearance of the sinus are characteristic in that there is a moderate reduction in the translucency of **all** the sinuses. Only if there is supper-added infection are dense opacity or fluid levels seen on X-ray.

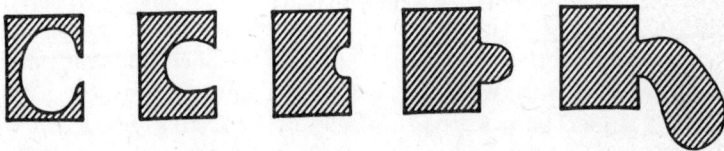

Fig. 23. Left: The ethmoid cell with normal lining. The next four diagrams show how increasing swelling of the lining leads to protrusion of the lining out of the sinus into the lumen of airspace.

A **therapeutic trial** with various anti-allergic medicaments may be helpful in establishing the diagnosis. A clinical reponse to antihistamines or topically applied steroid such as Beconase (beclomethason dipropionate) is strong evidence in favour of an allergic basis for the patient's symptoms.

In the past, it was thought that **skin-testing** would provide useful evidence of a direct cause and effect relationship between a challenge with various allergens and the clinical reponse. Unfortunately, because most allergic patients tend to react positively to most allergens these tests are no longer considered of much practical assistance in diagnosis or treatment.

Treatment

The treatment of nasal allergy tends to be a complicated and long drawn out process, but with perseverance the condition of most patients can be improved. Of the two main forms of nasal allergy, the treatment of **seasonal allergy** is, as a rule, more satisfactory. To some extent this can be achieved **by avoidance** and many patients are able to diminish their symptoms in this way. Although antihistamines may reduce the severity of the symptoms, most patients are assisted most by hyposensitization. Two injections, at an interval of one week, of an aqueous suspension of the common local pollen allergens are given during the month of March.

The treatment of **perennial nasal allergy** is usually less satisfactory, largely due to the multiplicity and wide distribution of nasal allergens.

Treatment begins with limiting as far as possible exposure to all the common allergens. Success may depend upon such radical measures as changing jobs or dispensing with domestic pets. Because house dust, and particularly one of its constituents, the dust mite, is an important cause of perennial allergy, feather pillows and duvets should be replaced by non-allergic man-made alternatives. Mattresses should be vacuum-cleaned frequently and enclosed in plastic. When necessary, the dimensions of the nasal airways should be restored surgically by correcting septal deflections, removing polypi, and reducing the bulk of hypertrophic inferior turbinates. Indeed, to be effective, treatment must often **start** with the correction of anatomical defects so that the normal airflow patterns essential for nasal health can be re-established. Concurrent sinus infection must be sought and eliminated not only because it inevitably worsens the symptoms but also because the patient may eventually develop an allergic response to his own bacteria.

Temporary and limited symptomatic control may be obtained by antihistamines such as Fabahistin (mebhydrolin), Actifed (triprolidine hydrochloride; pseudoephedrine hydrochloride), or Histryl (diphenylpyraline hydrochloride), but some patients find these drugs unacceptable because of the soporific effect. Rynacrom (sodium cromoglycate) as a spray limits the release of histamine by preventing the degranulation of mast cells, and various steroid preparations such as Bextasol (betamethasone valerate) and Beconase (beclomethasone dipropionate) frequently provide relief, but again, their effect is symptomatic and certainly not curative. Fortunately, many sufferers from perennial rhinitis can now be significantly improved on the longer term by the use of mite-fortified house-dust vaccine. Although the durability of the results of this therapy is not yet known, there is evidence that significant improvements can be expected, if once-monthly maintenance injections are continued for several years.

It should be noted that the prolonged use of nasal drops containing ephedrine is to be deplored and must be warned against, because of their eventual damaging effect on the nasal mucosa (rhinitis medicamentosa).

It should be emphasized that the control of perennial nasal allergy is usually short of perfect, especially in our twentieth century environment of air pollution and inadequately humidified air-conditioning.

NASAL INFECTION

This may be acute and of short duration as in coryza and influenza, or persistent, when those conditions fail to resolve in the usual way. Nasal allergy and anatomic abnormalities predispose to chronicity and the condition is often complicated and perpetuated by sinusitis and bronchitis. Nasal foreign bodies in children also cause infection which is usually unilateral.

Symptoms

Nasal obstruction is due to inflammatory swelling of the mucosa and the presence of viscous secretions in the nasal cavity. Nose-blowing will produce mucus initially and then mucopus, and the voice will have a 'nasal' quality. With coryza, headache, loss of appetite, sore throat and malaise will frequently occur during the first few days.

Diagnosis

The diagnosis of nasal infection will usually be reached on the evidence of the history and in the chronic type after exclusion of uncomplicated anatomic obstruction, allergy, and concomitant sinus infection as the primary causes of the above symptoms.

In acute nasal infections, pyrexia is often present initially: in the chronic state it should suggest the possibility of complications such as sinusitis, otitis media, or bronchopneumonia.

Clinical presentation

In the *acute form,* the patient is hot and flushed and appears to be unwell. He will be mouth-breathing, and mucopus may be seen in the nose and on the posterior wall of the pharynx.

In the *chronic form,* the patient looks less ill and may often be back at work. However, he also will be mouth-breathing and there will usually be infected secretions to be seen in his nose and on his handkerchief.

Treatment

In the **acute phase,** confinement to bed in a warm, humid atmosphere with plentiful fluids and aspirin gr. 10 three times daily, will often suffice.

Nasal decongestion can be promoted topically by ephedrine drops or systemically with Actified Compound Linctus (triprolidine hydrochloride; pseudoephedrine hydrochloride; codeine phosphate) 1 ml (¼-teaspoonful) three times daily for children, 5–10 ml three times daily for adults — the dose for each to be regulated in regard to need and to the degree of sedation produced. Complications should be dealt with on their merits.

Normally, the disease lasts for one to two weeks, by which time normal activity should gradually be resumed.

In the **chronic phase,** a cause of failure for the acute phase to resolve as expected should be sought and dealt with. Polypi may require removal or an infected maxillary antrum need irrigation. Antiallergic and antibacterial treatment will often be essential to secure a successful outcome, and this will be assisted by light exercise in fresh air when climatic conditions are favourable.

When the cause of chronic unilateral purulent nasal discharge is found to be a foreign body (usually in children), treatment consists of removal, as described in chapter 18 (page 123) of this book.

ANATOMICAL ABNORMALITIES

These include deflections of the nasal septum, hypertrophy of the middle and inferior turbinates, and adenoidal enlargement.

Deviated nasal septum is usually the result of trauma but apparently occurs, though rarely, as a genetic trait. Even a minor injury in early childhood can result in major septal deformity in later life owing to the fact that the mutual influence on the development of each bone by its neighbour is altered during the growth phase. Obstruction to breathing is due not only to a physical reduction of air space but also and often more significantly to turbulence arising from disturbance of the normal air current pathways.

Treatment is surgical by the submucous resection operation (SMR) which is performed under general anaesthesia and entails a four- to five-day period in hospital.

Hypertrophic turbinates are practically always allergic in origin. They are a major source of excess mucus production in allergic rhinitis and they certainly detract from nasal health by their interference with airflow patterns.

Their bulk can be reduced by a combination of submucosal diathermy and judicial trimming under general anaesthesia, especially when, as is frequently the case in allergy, there is hypertrophy of the posterior ends of the inferior turbinates. In addition to widening the airways, these procedures will frequently reduce the amount of mucus secretion by reducing the numbers of secreting glands.

Adenoidal enlargement is the most common cause of nasal obstruction in the young and follows recurrent nasopharyngeal infection. Once established, adenoid enlargement rarely subsides spontaneously and if allowed to persist will lead to the development of the 'adenoidal facies' — stupid expression, mouth-breathing, high-arched palate, and prominent upper teeth — and will frequently be complicated by recurrent otitis media and sinusitis.

'Adenoids' as the cause of nasal obstruction in children will require specialist examination to differentiate it from nasal allergy and deviation of the nasal septum. However, as indicated, nasal obstruction in the young can cause far-reaching impairment of health and therefore referral to an ENT clinic is always indicated for this symptom, regardless of the cause, should it fail to respond promptly to medication with decongestant mixtures such as Actifed Compound Linctus (triprolidine hydrochloride; pseudoephedrine hydrochloride; codeine phosphate).

The diagnosis of enlarged adenoids is confirmed by mirror examination (in the co-operative child), the inference that large tonsils usually indicate a large adenoid mass, and by lateral X-rays of the postnasal space.

From the above, it will be obvious that this condition should not be neglected. Unfortunately, medical treatment by antibacterial substances or decongestants is rarely successful — fortunately, removal of the adenoid mass by curettage under general anaesthesia is curative.

Summary

The treatment of the blocked or persistently discharging nose is never an easy matter. It is most important to realize that the patient's condition may be complicated by the co-existence of various abnormalities and that symptoms such as nasal obstruction and hypersecretion may be contributed to by anatomical problems, the presence of infection, by dysfunction of the endocrine system, and even by inherent vasomotor instability as occurs in the elderly. Although in many cases allergy is the basic cause of 'catarrh', other factors should always be suspected and should certainly be dealt with as far as possible before specific anti-allergic treatment is commenced.

REVISION: CAUSES OF NASAL OBSTRUCTION

For revision purposes, the chief causes of nasal obstruction can be classified as follows:

1. **Congenital** posterior choanal atresia

2. **Traumatic**
   (a) septal haematoma
   (b) deviated nasal septum

3. **Inflammatory**
   (a) vestibulary furunculosis
   (b) septal abscess
   (c) coryza and influenza
   (d) sinusitis
   (e) nasal allergy
   (f) non-specific vasomotor rhinitis
   (g) nasal polypi
   (h) foreign body

4. **Neoplastic**
   (a) benign
       (i) fibroma
       (ii) angioma and angiofibroma

      (iii) chondroma
      (iv) osteoma
   (b) malignant
      (i) carcinoma
      (ii) adenocarcinoma
      (iii) melanoma
      (iv) Wegener's granuloma
      (v) mixed salivary tumour
      (vi) cylindroma

5. **Others**
   (a) hormonal
   (b) rhinitis medicamentosa
   (c) reserpine type drugs

10. Headache and facial pain

Although many patients who suffer from headaches or facial pain begin their first consultation with the statement that they are suffering from 'sinusitis', in reality this does not always prove to be the case. The sensory innervation of the area is mainly trigeminal, a complex, intercommunicating system which is characterized by its predilection for apparent erroneous reporting due actually to variable thresholds, summation, and other neurogenic phenomena which are the basis of referred pain. Consequently, pain which appears to be originating from the sinuses may have a quite different source. The patient's misinterpretation of his problem is often supported by concomitant nasal stuffiness due to an associated reflex engorgement of the nasal mucosa.

Although sinus infection is a frequent cause of facial pain and headache, the possible existence of intracranial causes, the various form of migraine, trigeminal neuralgia, temporal arteritis, and referred pain from lesions of the masticatory apparatus must always be considered carefully.

As is usual in ENT practice, a well-elicited history will generally give a clear lead to the probable diagnosis.

SINUSITIS

Practically all sinus infection is a complication of nasal infection (exceptions are those which originate from an upper molar tooth abscess or penetrating injury). Therefore, a history of recent coryza and concurrent infected nasal symptoms are almost essential for the diagnosis. Again, the duration, location, and time cycle of the headache is important to the diagnosis. In distinction to headaches from other sources, the onset of headache in sinusitis is closely related to the development of symptoms of nasal infection; pain is usually unilateral and frontal, and tends to be most severe in the first few hours after waking, diminishing or even disappearing from early afternoon until the next day. The patient looks and feels ill with pyrexia 38–39 °C; 100–102 °F). Mucopus in the nose (or on the handkerchief) or seen trickling down the posterior wall of the pharynx strongly supports the diagnosis which is confirmed by the results of transillumination and X-ray, and finally, if need be, by proof puncture of the appropriate maxillary antrum.

Treatment

The patient can usually be bed-nursed at home in a warm, humidified atmosphere, and prompt treatment with appropriate antimicrobials — Penbritin (ampicillin) or Septrin (trimethoprim; sulphamethoxazole) — combined with oral decongestants — Actifed Compound Linctus (triprolidine hydrochloride; pseudoephedrine hydrochloride) — ephedrine nose drops, analgesics as required, and a light fluid diet, will control most sinus infections within a few days. However, should there be failure to respond, i.e. should temperature elevation persist, pain worsen, or should there be evidence of extending infection (orbital cellulitis, frontal swelling, etc) then drainage of the affected sinus as an in-patient measure under general anaesthesia is urgently required.

Virtually all sinusitis involves the antrum primarily, and adequate treatment of this sinus will usually be followed by recovery of associated frontal and ethmoidal infection.

Drainage of pus is achieved initially by antrum puncture and lavage, and treatment continued by repeated irrigation through indwelling polythene tubes until the return through the sinus ostium has been clear for 48 hours (Fig. 24). Supportive antibiotic therapy based on bacteriological studies will be given and complications arising from the formation of pus in the orbit or frontal sinus dealt with by appropriate drainage operations.

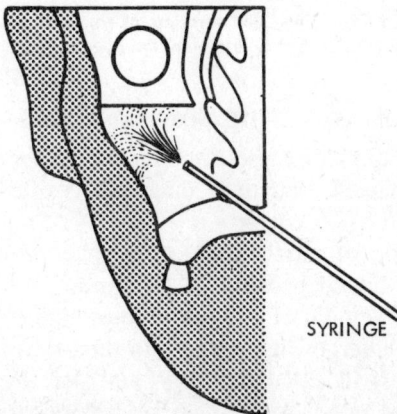

SYRINGE

Fig. 24. Following antral lavage with a trochar and cannula, further irrigations are performed through a polythene tube. This is passed into the antrum, using the cannula as a guide, and kept in position by strapping it to the skin of the nostril.

When acute maxillary sinusitis is neglected or unresponsive to treatment the cure of persistent facial pain, headache, and purulent nasal secretion will be beyond purely medical therapy, and will require surgical treatment aimed at long-term drainage of the antrum (intranasal antrostomy) (Fig. 25) or removal of chonically infected mucosa from the antrum (Caldwell–Luc operation), the ethmoids, or frontal sinus. In this situation, there is frequently an underlying allergic problem which will require continued specific treatment.

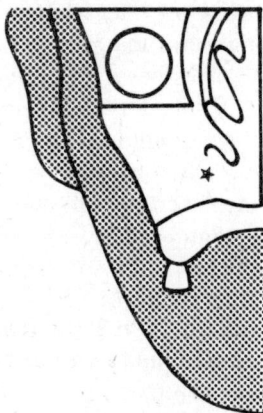

Fig. 25. Intranasal antrostomy. The removal of the medial antral wall inferior to the inferior turbinate (*) allows permanant drainage of the antrum into the nose.

MALIGNANT NEOPLASMS OF THE NOSE AND PARANASAL SINUSES

The early symptoms of these tumours are so similar to those of inflammatory disease that their diagnosis is often delayed until extensive spread has occurred.

After a period of nasal obstruction, mucopurulent discharge becomes blood-tinged because of ulceration, and pain develops because of involvement of sensory fibres of the trigeminal nerve. As the tumour enlarges, its spread into the orbit, the face, or the gums and palate, will lead to deformity and ulceration. Unexpected problems with an upper dental plate or diplopia are often the first signs of spread outside the sinus.

MALIGNANT NEOPLASMS OF THE POSTNASAL SPACE

These can involve the third to twelfth cranial nerves as they pass through their foramina in the base of the skull. Because tumours in this area will grow in different directions at different rates, the sequence of neural involvement is variable. Trigeminal neuropathy is frequent and results in severe facial pain whose distribution is related to the fibres affected.

HERPES ZOSTER

This virus infection can affect any of the sensory nerves in the area, especially the three branches of the trigeminal nerve and the nervus intermedius, the sensory branch of the seventh nerve, which relays afferent information from the skin of the external ear canal.

Pain in the distribution of the involved nerve is severe and usually precedes the vesicular skin eruption by four to seven days. After the rash has subsided it is not uncommon for pain to persist for months and, occasionally, years. Treatment with analgesics and steroids is usually recommended.

OTHER CAUSES OF HEADACHE AND FACIAL PAIN

The mechanism of headache from **intracranial disease** is often poorly understood. When it is due to a space-occupying lesion it is usually continuous, generalized, and increasingly severe. Neurological examination may provide evidence of motor or sensory deficit and increased intracranial pressure, and radiological investigation will frequently confirm the diagnosis.

Many patients who complain of 'sinusitis' actually suffer from **migraine** or one of its variants. This may be the textbook headache which is unilateral, periorbital, accompanied by nausea and photophobia, and preceded by an aura which the patient soon learns to recognize. More often the pain is more generalized, lasts many hours or even for several days, but characteristically the attacks tend to be clustered and often precipitated by stress. The diagnosis is frequently based on the exclusion of other causes and a positive response to the trial of ergot-containing drugs — Bellergal Retard (total alkaloids of belladonna; ergotamine tartrate; phenobarbitone) — or Dixarit (clonidine hydrochloride).

Trigeminal neuralgia gives rise to severe pain in the distribution of one of the branches of the fifth nerve and characteristically is triggered off by an oral stimulus such as eating or talking. In the absence of dental or ENT disease, the diagnosis is confirmed by a positive response to treatment with Tegretol (carbamazepine).

In **temporal arteritis,** pain radiates from the area of distribution of the superficial temporal artery which is usually visibly convoluted and tender on palpation. The diagnosis is confirmed by biopsy and marked elevation of the erythrocyte sedimentation rate. Steroid therapy is usually curative and prevents ocular complications.

'Sinusitis' and **abnormalities of the masticatory apparatus** are often confused by patient and doctor alike. Pain in this condition is due to spasm of one or all of the pterygoid, masseter, or temporalis muscles, and is frequently severe and persistent, and as with the migrainous neuralgias, can be recurrent for years. Stress is an aggravating factor which often leads to jaw-clamping and teeth-grinding in patients with skew jaw movement and 'over-bite' and in those who wear dentures which fit poorly. In such patients, a dramatic cure can usually be achieved through correction of the jaw abnormality by an oral surgeon with understanding of these problems.

Dental infection. Although dental abscess is rarely responsible for headache, it is a frequent cause of facial pain and also for pain referred to those othere areas which are innervated by the sensory fibres of the fifth cranial nerve. Once other causes have been excluded, referral for appropriate dental treatment is called for.

REVISION: CAUSES OF HEADACHE AND FACIAL PAIN

For revision purposes, the chief causes of headache are classified as follows:

1. **Traumatic**
   (a) head injury
   (b) fractured facial bones

2. **Inflammatory**
   (a) infections of the scalp and skin
   (b) preauricular adenitis
   (c) vestibular funculosis
   (d) acute sinusitis and its complications
   (e) dental infection
   (f) erysipelas
   (g) herpes
   (h) temporal arteritis
   (i) orbital infections
   (j) infections of the petrous apex

11. Nasal haemorrhage

Epistaxis occurs most commonly in the young and is due to trauma or infection — usually coryza. It may be associated with measles or influenza or arise as a complication of haemopoietic disease.

In young persons bleeding from the anterior part of the nasal septum (Fig. 26) can usually be controlled by compressing the

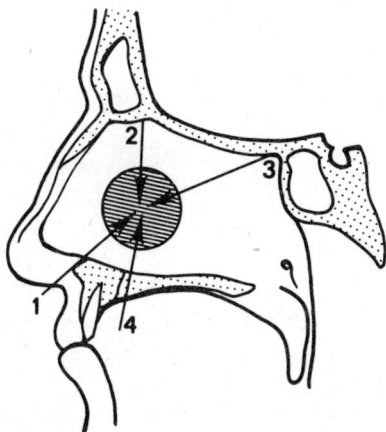

Fig. 26. The anterior part of the nasal septum (Little's area) is fed by the superior labial artery (1), the anterior ethmoidal artery (2), and the septal (3) and descending palatine (4) branches of the sphenopalatine arteries.

nostrils for a few minutes, assisted by the application of cold packs to the face and neck to produce reflex vasoconstriction (Fig. 27). Failing this, a plug of wool or a length of half-inch ribbon gauze inserted well into the nose will usually terminate the bleeding, at least temporarily. Should epistaxis persist or recur, a more permanent solution can be achieved by chemical or electrocautery of the bleeding vessels using local anaesthesia (Fig. 28).

Epistaxis **in the middle-aged and elderly** may have serious connotations because of its frequent association with arteriosclerosis and hypertension. Certain branches of the internal maxillary artery enter the nasal cavity far back and in so doing turn forwards

3. **Neoplastic**
   (a) malignant tumours of the nose, sinuses, postnasal space, middle ear, and orbit
   (b) acoustic neurinoma, and other intracranial neoplasms

4. **Others**
   (a) disorders of the temperomandibular joint and jaws
   (b) trigeminal neuralgia
   (c) migraine

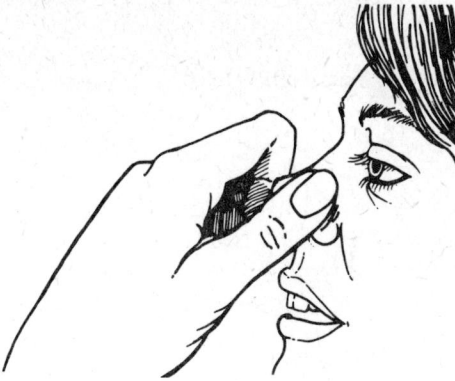

Fig. 27.

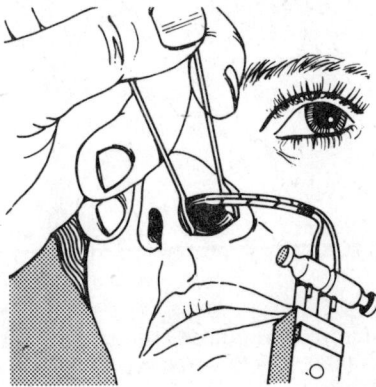

Fig. 28.

through an angle of 90°. If, at this angle, there is an atheromatous area, then at any time a sudden elevation of blood pressure in conjunction with inflammation due to upper respiratory infection may lead to profuse haemorrhage which, because of the poor contractability of atheromatous vessels is likely to persist, with life-threatening results.

Hospital treatment: when there is profuse bleeding, transfer to a hospital ENT department is usually advisable. There, it will be possible to clean and anaesthetize the nose so as to identify the source of bleeding more accurately and control it either by cautery, if the vessel is accessible, or by the application of pressure from (i) accurately placed packs of half-inch gauze impregnated in bismuth iodoform paraffin paste (BIPP) (Fig. 29), or (ii) an inflatable rubber bag.

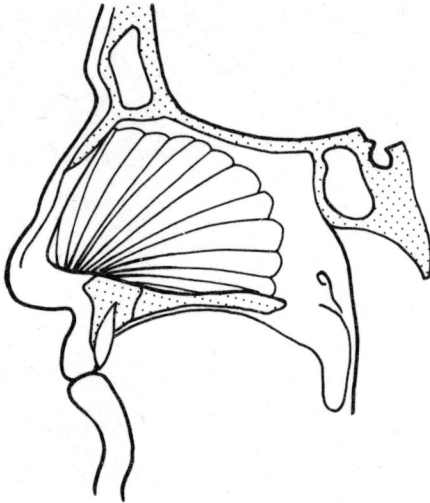

Fig. 29. After anaesthetizing the nose with a Lignocaine spray, a pack of half-inch gauze is built up, layer upon layer, between the floor and the roof of the nasal cavity.

If packing the nose is required, the patient should be admitted to the ENT ward so that any necessary blood replacement and general supportive measures against shock can be carried out. The packs will be left undisturbed under antibiotic cover until secure thrombosis of the affected vessels has occurred, which will take several days. Should repeated nasal packing be unsuccessful, then ligation of the appropriate artery, i.e. the anterior ethmoidal, external carotid, or internal maxillary, may be required.

During hospitalization, the general state of the patient's health, with especial references to cardiovascular and haemolytic disease, should be investigated and treated appropriately.

Facial trauma is a common cause of epistaxis which usually ceases spontaneously although recovery may often be hastened by the application of cold compresses to the head and neck. Concomitant displacement of the nasal bones, maxilla, or zygoma may require manipulation under general anaesthetic and temporary support with splints. If septal haematoma complicates the injury and causes nasal obstruction, this should be treated by incision or aspiration to avoid abscess formation.

REVISION: CAUSES AND TREATMENT OF NASAL HAEMORRAGE

The causes are:

1. **Local**
   (a) coryza
   (b) trauma
   (c) malignancy
   (d) foreign body
   (e) telangiectasis

2. **General**
   (a) prodromal stages of infectious disease
   (b) blood dyscrasias
   (c) hypertension
   (d) drugs

The principles of treatment are:

1. Stop the bleeding

2. Replace blood loss when necessary.

3. Treat the cause.

The throat

12. Anatomy and physiology

The throat has two parts — the pharynx and the larynx.

The pharynx
The pharynx forms the upper end of the digestive tract and partici-
pates in swallowing, respiration, and vocalization. It extends from
the base of the skull to the cricoid cartilage in three parts (Fig. 30):

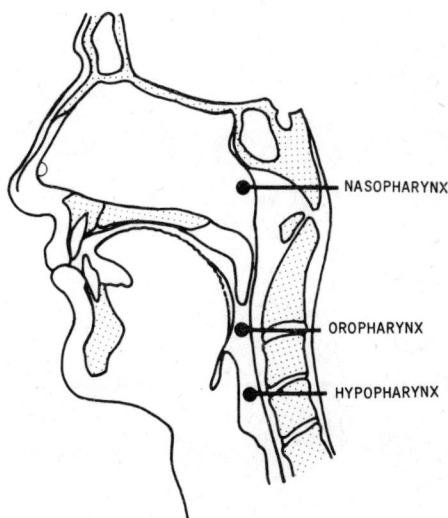

Fig. 30.

(1) **the nasopharynx,** communicating anteriorly with the nasal
cavity and laterally via the Eustachian tube with the tympanum,
and inferiorly with

(2) **the oropharynx,** which extends from the soft palate above
to the larynx below, and communicates anteriorly with the buccal
cavity through the pillars of the fauces, and

(3) **the hypopharynx** which surrounds the larynx laterally and
posteriorly and leads into the upper end of the oesophagus.

The walls of the pharynx are an incomplete muscular sleeve
mostly lined by squamous epithelium.

Aggregates of lymph tissue lie in the subepithelium of the naso-pharynx (adenoid), between the pillars of the fauces (palatine tonsil) and across the base of the tongue (lingual tonsil).

The adenoid occupies the vault of the nasopharynx and extends laterally, posterior to the orifice of the Eustachian tube. Its surface is corrugated and covered by ciliated epithelium.

The palatine and lingual tonsils are covered by squamous epithe-lium. They vary greatly in size and the surface is rendered irregular by the orifices of crypts which extend deeply into their substance.

The lymphoid tissue of the tonsils and adenoid (Waldeyer's ring) (Fig. 31) is arranged in follicles which drain, by lymphatic channels, into the upper deep cervical lymph nodes. Their mass is minimal at birth, maximal between five to ten years, and then slowly atrophies. This applies especially to the adenoid which is often absent by 12 years.

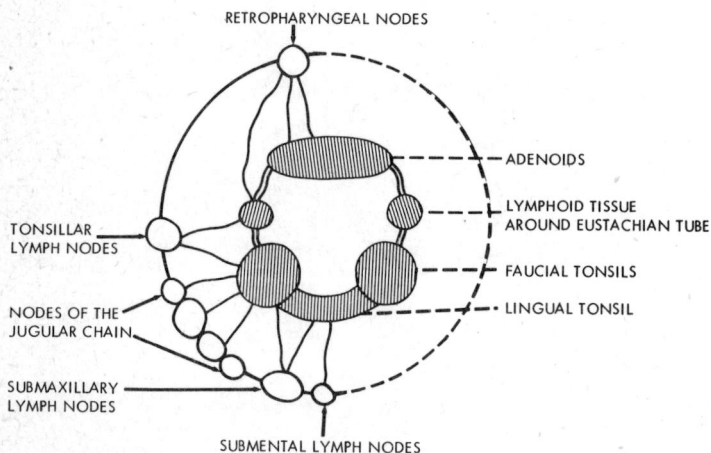

Fig. 31. Waldeyer's ring.

The function of the tonsils and adenoid, especially in early life, is protective through the localization of infection and the produc-tion of antibodies.

The larynx

The larynx passes antero-inferiorly from the oropharynx, and lies in front of the hypopharynx. It protects the lower respiratory tract and transmits air for respiration and vocalization.

The larynx is a membrano-cartilaginous tube whose oriface is controlled by the aryepiglottic folds which protect the lungs by their sphincteric action, and shielded by the leaf-like epiglottis. The diaphragm and thoracic cage act as a bellows which creates an airflow through the larynx. This flow is regulated by fibrous bands covered with squamous epithelium, which project into its lumen (the vocal cords). Alteration in the position and tension of the cords produce variations in the rate and volume of air flow and convert it into a vibratory column. In this way, sound is produced which can then be modulated and given resonance by the pharynx, palate, tongue, mouth, lips, and sinuses, thus giving rise to voice.

13. Sore throat

Presentation

When a patient complains of sore throat it is frequently possible to predict the diagnosis from the history and your observations of him as you take that history — so always, as you question and listen to the answers, observe how the patient looks, note his age group, the health of his complexion, etc. Always ask yourself whether his general state appears to be more in line with an inflammatory disease or a malignant one.

Remember that sore throat lasting for more than a few weeks in a middle-aged or elderly patient strongly suggests the possibility of malignancy. This is likely when there is difficulty in swallowing solids or hoarseness. A history of 'something in the throat', 'a crumb', or a feeling of a 'lump' in the throat extending back for several years in a female patient now complaining of recent persistent sore throat suggests that a post-cricoid carcinoma has complicated a pre-existing Patterson, Brown–Kelly syndrome. The patient's life-style may be relevant to the symptoms and enquiry should be made into the possibility of trauma from excessively hot food or drink, vocal abuse, or over-consumption of tobacco (even five cigarettes daily may cause sore throat in certain susceptible individuals).

Appropriate questions should be asked to detect such causes of sore throat as vitamin C deficiency, leukaemia, hiatus hernia, or associated chronic sinusitis. Recent antibiotic therapy should raise the suspicion of *Candida* infection.

Although full examination of the pharynx is only possible after specialist training in the use of headlight, spatula, and angled mirrors, nevertheless, it is often possible to obtain valuable information by examination of the oropharynx and nose using a good torch and wooden tongue depressor combined with palpation of the neck.

If, after this, the cause of sore throat is not immediately apparent, then referral to an ENT specialist is urgently required.

The painful conditions of the oropharynx which can be detected by non-specialist examination will now be discussed. These can be divided into inflammatory and neoplastic disease. All those practising medicine should have some knowledge about the appearances and treatment of these conditions, both because they are common and also because many are usually best-treated at once by those who first diagnose them rather than wait until a hospital appointment can be arranged.

The characteristic 'diagnostic' symptoms of conditions not identified by simple examination of the oropharynx will also be discussed in regard to significant aspects of the history, which, if recognized for their worth, will prompt expedient referral to an ENT clinic.

ACUTE INFLAMMATORY CONDITIONS OF THE OROPHARYNX

Acute pharyngitis is the result of infection by either viruses or bacteria. All age groups are susceptible but the highest incidence is in childhood and peaks of infection occur in September, January, and March.

Initial symptoms

1. In **virus infections,** e.g. rhinovirus, adenovirus, parainfluenza, and influenza, the initial symptoms include nasal stuffiness, water nasal discharge, and nasopharyngeal discomfort. Within 24–48 hours, sore throat is added to these. The development of purulent secretions suggests secondary bacterial infection.

2. In **bacterial pharyngitis,** e.g. streptococci, staphylococci, pneumococci, and *Haemophilus influenzae,* sore throat, often initially unilateral, advances rapidly. (NB: In bacterial infections, sore throat causes much more distress than nasal symptoms in the early stages. This is not the case in viral infections.)

Course

From that stage onwards, both viral and bacterial infections run a similar course. The symptoms include increasing discomfort on swallowing even to the point of inability to swallow saliva, malaise, and headache. The temperature is elevated (38–40°C; 100–104°F) and on examination there is increasing hyperaemia of the palate, the uvula (which may be swollen), and the oropharyngeal mucosa (with prominence of lymph follicles on the posterior pharyngeal wall) and if the tonsils are present they will become swollen and grossly inflamed. Purulent exudate may be seen in the orifices of the crypts or even cover the tonsillar surface. There will be enlargement and tenderness of the glands below the angle of the jaw (jugulo-digastric). Usually, symptoms persist from one to two weeks. Acute otitis media, sinusitis, tracheitis, laryngitis, and bronchitis may occur as complications. Occasionally, infection may penetrate the tonsillar capsule to form a peritonsillar abscess (quinsy), when, in addition to the effects of tonsillar infection, the patient will have difficulty in opening his mouth (trismus) due to spasm of the masticatory muscles. If the mouth can be opened enough it will be seen that a swelling in the outer part of the soft palate has displaced the tonsil and uvula towards the other side.

Treatment

Antibiotics and sulphonamides are not beneficial to the patient in uncomplicated viral infections. Thus, acute pharyngitis of viral origin should be treated **initially** by:

(a) bed rest in a humidifed atmosphere;

(b) light fluid diet;

(c) nasal decongestion by half per cent ephedrine drops four-hourly, and Actifed Compound Linctus (triprolidine hydro-chloride; pseudoephedrine hydrochloride; codeine phosphate) (dosage appropriate to age); and

(d) aspirin for its symptomatic effect.

However, if there is evidence of acute tonsillitis or otitis media, on the assumption that bacterial infection is imminent, if not already present, then treatment is augmented by the addition of antibiotic (having first taken a throat swab so that the initial choice of antibiotic can be adjusted in regard to sensitivity, should there be a failure of clinical response). The drug of choice is ampicillin. The dosage in children is 250 mg eight-hourly and in adults, 500 mg eight-hourly, for at least five days. When quinsy does not respond rapidly to this treatment, prompt relief will follow incision of the abscess where it projects superolaterally to the tonsil.

RECURRENT INFECTIONS OF THE OROPHARYNX

Recurrent pharyngitis can be troublesome in all age groups and required separate consideration.

It most frequently occurs in those who still retain their tonsils and the condition is essentially recurrent acute tonsillitis. In these patients, the basic health of the tonsil is usually defective, from

failure completely to resolve previous infections, with resultant scarring and chronic abscess formation within the tonsil. The stability of such an organ is tenuous and easily upset by assaults which the healthy tonsil would parry without difficulty, such as from relatively small numbers of pathogenic bacteria in the presence of reduced body temperature due to wet feet, hair-washing or even standing briefly in a cold draught, or irritants such as tobacco smoke or alcohol.

The treatment of recurrent tonsillitis is related to the age of the patient. The solution to the problem up to the age of about 12 is quite different from that in older people.

Childhood tonsillitis

It has been shown that during the first decades of life, children who suffer from recurrent bouts of tonsillitis have significant immuno-deficiencies. The tonsils in health are an important source of total body immunoglobulin. Obviously the contribution of the unhealthy tonsil must be less than normal.

Ideally, treatment should prevent further loss of normal tonsillar tissue with preservation and functional improvement of the residuum. The traditional method of therapy in children is dissection of the tonsil but this removes both the tissue which is the site of recurrent infections, and that which contributes to the fight against infection. Although tonsillectomy will usually reduce the incidence of pharyngitis in the immediate postoperative years, it may also cause a weakening of the patient's overall resistance and is undoubtedly attended by a long list of complications which, although not common, are significant and include psychological disturbances and a small but tragic mortality.

Public — and much medical — opinion frequently has it that tonsils should be removed because they are large. Unless their size is causing an irreversible and dangerous obstruction to breathing or swallowing, which is extremely rare, their removal on the grounds of size is illogical. Large tonsils are usually busy tonsils — busy in the production of antibody, a work in which they should be encouraged. Although many children suffer from frequent acute tonsillitis during the first few years of school life, they do not all necessarily require tonsillectomy as the *first* means of treatment. Many can be treated with considerable success by long-term anti-bacterial therapy which will diminish the frequency of repetitive attacks of acute infection, prevent further destruction of the tonsil, and at the same time, allow the remaining tonsillar tissue to regain its health and resume its role of antibody formation.

Thus, during the first decade, every effort should be made to preserve the tonsil (and to avoid the risks and expense of removal) for as long as the frequency of tonsillitis can be controlled. This can often be done by continuous treatment with such agents as Penicillin V (phenoxymethylpenicillin) or Septrin (trimethoprim sulphamethoxazole), given in courses of not less than three months (which can be repeated once or twice each year if required), with appropriate reassessments of the history and health of the tonsils. Thus, many young children are brought back to health and spared an unnecessary operation. However, should such a regime fail to limit the frequency of acute tonsillitis to one or two attacks per year, then it must be recognized without further ado that conservative treatment has failed and tonsillectomy and adenoidectomy are now indicated.

Older children and adults

After age 12, the situation is quite different. By this time prior recurrent attacks of tonsillitis will have caused destruction of much functional tonsillar tissue which has been replaced by scar tissue and lymphatic granulomata. The ability and indeed the need of the tonsil to produce antibodies is by now much reduced so that retention of this chronically infected focus offers little advantage and may often be deleterious to health. Such tonsils are small and fibrotic; pus or debris, sometimes both, can often be expressed from their crypts; and the continuance of infection within the tonsil can be deduced from the observed congestion of blood vessels causing a red flush along the anterior tonsillar pillar.

The period of urgent antibody production has been passed; the tonsil is no longer contributing to that cause and is indeed now the source of recurrent spread of infection into nearby areas, in particular the pharynx — at this stage antibacterial therapy proves unhelpful and solution of the problem is best achieved by surgical removal of the burnt-out, permanently infected organ. After the age of 12, the morbidity and mortality are practically negligible and the success rate in terms of preventing recurrent pharyngitis is so high that tonsillectomy is now usually indicated.

Summary: recommended treatment for recurrent acute tonsillitis
1. When the attacks last five to seven days and occur more than four times a year for two or more years:

(a) in young children, initially long-term treatment with anti-bacterial agents should be instigated in an attempt to sterilize the tonsil and thus restore its health and ability to function;

(b) in children where continued medical treatment proves unsuccessful, and in all patients over 12 years of age, tonsillectomy will be necessary to restore the health of the oropharynx.

2. Tonsillectomy will usually be necessary:

(a) when chronic infection of the tonsil (pus expressed from the crypts, or persistent inflammatory enlargement with palpable tonsillar lymph glands) causes persistent or recurrent pharyngitis;

(b) when there has been a previous quinsy;

(c) when tonsils carry virulent organisms not necessarily associated with symptoms:

(i) in hospital personnel posing the threat of infection in their patients and colleagues;

(ii) in patients who have carditis or nephritis.

CHRONIC IRRITATION OF THE PHARYNX

Again, the duration and character of the symptoms will suggest the diagnosis. Chronic pharyngitis is a disease of adult life in which the complaint is of persistent discomfort rather than acute pain. The condition may be perpetuated by infection of the nasal sinuses, or dental apparatus, or associated with chronically infected tonsils, chronic bronchitis, or bronchiectasis. Not infrequently, it is the result of chronic mouth-breathing due to nasal obstruction caused by septal deflection or allergy. Faulty voice production, the inhalation of industrial fumes, central heating lacking proper humidification, over-use of tobacco and alcohol, and the consumption of very hot or spicy food, should always be evaluated as possible perpetuating factors.

The length of the history is important to the diagnosis. When symptoms may have been present continuously or intermittently for several years before advice is sought, chronic inflammatory (but not necessarily infectious) causes are likely. After taking the history, inspection of the oropharynx will confirm the diagnosis. The mucosa is thickened and engorged with increased mucus secretion which may form a thick film over the posterior wall of the pharynx. As a rule, the lymphatic pharyngeal lymph tissue is hypertrophied, raising prominent vertical red bands of tissue laterally and giving the posterior wall a rough granular (Morocco leather) appearance.

Chronic sepsis of the nose and gums, and the presence of mouth-breathing should be noted. As always, it is important to consider the patient as a whole because chronic pharyngitis occasionally presents as a complication of diseases such as nephritis, cirrhosis, or cardiac insufficiency.

Treatment

1. **Control related chronic sepsis** appropriately.
2. **Correct defects of the nasal airway** by surgical means followed by retraining in nasal breathing.
3. Large aggregates of granular lymphatic tissue in the pharynx may require reduction by **cryosurgery or galvanocautery.**
4. An important part of treatment consists of explaining the mechanism of chronic pharyngitis to the patient so that he can attempt to correct the inevitable perpetuating factors in his **life style.** This may involve changing his job to avoid industrial fumes, undergoing a course in speech training, regulating his dietary habits or his consumption of alcohol and tobacco. The patient must understand the importance of ceasing the continuous coughing, hawking, and throat-clearing which is characteristic of the condition.
5. **Medication:**
    (a) To reduce the viscosity of the mucus secretion, oily nasal drops containing white paraffin (one part) and liquid paraffin (three parts) or Argyrol nasal drops 10% in saline solution are often helpful. Alternatively, the quality of the mucus secretion may be improved by the ingestion of Organidin Elixir (iodinated glyceryl; alcohol) 5 ml three times daily for one month.
    (b) To remove excessive amounts of sticky mucus physically, a bland gargle such as normal saline or glycothymoline at body temperature, should be prescribed. Ferriperchlorate solution used as a gargle several times daily over a period of weeks has an improving effect on hypertrophic mucosa. Note that gargles containing irritant substances such as phenol should be avoided because although they may provide temporary symptomatic relief, they are likely to aggravate the condition.

It should be emphasized that antibiotic therapy has no part in the treatment of chronic pharyngitis, except in those patients where there is a clearly defined focus of sepsis in which case they may be given with effect in conjunction with the appropriate surgical procedure.

Pharyngitis due to gastric reflux

A significant number of patients suffer from chronic sore throat because of the effects of gastric reflux with or without hiatus hernia. The patient is often overweight and often female. Symptoms may date from the last pregnancy: heartburn at night or indigestion is frequent. The symptoms are due to chronic irritation of the mucosa and inco-ordination of the cricopharyngeal sphincter. The Patterson, Brown–Kelly syndrome is associated with hypochromic anaemia, angular stomatitis, koilonychia, and often monilial infection. Barium studies must be augmented by direct examination under anaesthesia to establish the diagnosis and rule out malignancy.

The treatment of this type of pharyngitis is as for hiatus hernia with maintenance of normal blood and serum iron levels. Periodic and continued observation is necessary because there is a risk of eventual postcricoid carcinoma when this condition is inadequately treated.

MALIGNANCY IN THE OROPHARYNX

Pain is frequently preceded by an abnormal sensation and patients will often complain initially of a feeling of 'something in the throat' or that a crumb is caught there and cannot be shifted. At this stage a tumour in the oropharynx will be seen as a smooth mass arising from the tonsillar area or from the base of the tongue, but eventually most become ulcerated and give rise to pain on swallowing.

When sore throat lasts for more than two weeks, any pharyngeal ulcer should be considered potentially malignant until proven otherwise by biopsy, as a hospital out-patient procedure. The presence of non-painful enlargement of the upper deep cervical glands is highly suggestive of carcinoma or reticulosarcoma somewhere in the upper respiratory tract. Once the diagnosis has been confirmed by biopsy, treatment will usually be by surgery, radiotherapy, and cytotoxic drugs as appropriate to the site, nature, and extent of the tumour.

So far, we have been concerned with causes of sore throat which can be identified by simple examination of the throat with a torch and spatula. Because there are areas of the pharynx which require more sophisticated methods of examination, whenever the cause of sore throat is not readily elucidated by simple spatular examination, the condition should at once be regarded as potentially serious and urgent referral made to an ENT clinic. This is because the symptoms of chronic pharyngitis due to gastric reflux and those of malignant tumours are so similar, and also because chronic inflammation of the hypopharynx has a malign tendency.

As a rule, carcinoma of the hypopharynx occurs in the pyriform sinus in males and in the postcricoid region in females. The early symptoms, which are similar to those caused by tumours of the oropharynx, are often vague and tend to be neglected until pain or difficulty in swallowing supervenes. At this stage the tumour is ulcerated, extensive, and involves the lymph nodes.

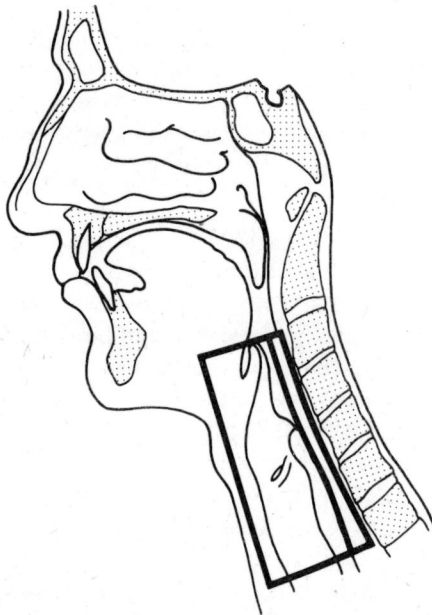

Fig. 32. The area of tissue to be excised in total laryngectomy and laryngopharyngectomy (larger box) is indicated.

The diagnosis is based on suspicion of throat symptoms in all over the age of 30, and confirmed by direct examination under anaesthetic with biopsy.

Treatment

Treatment is initially with radiotherapy. When this fails then radical surgery to remove the tumour and its associated lymph nodes, often with radiotherapy is necessary (Figs 32 and 33).

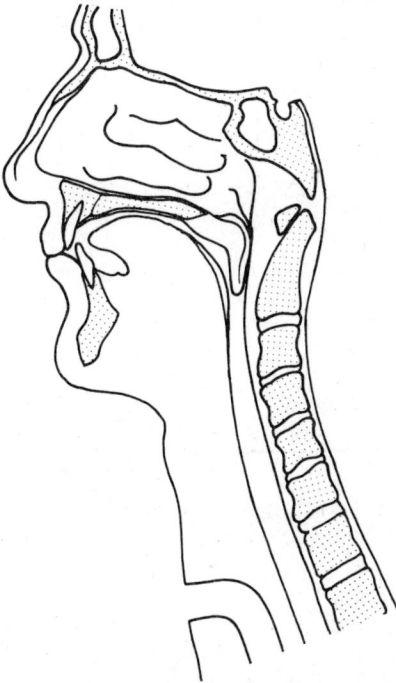

Fig. 33. The remaining pharyngeal mucosa and musculature is used to reconstruct the pharynx. The upper end of the trachea is brought to the surface of the neck.

REVISION: CAUSES OF SORE THROAT

For revision purposes, the chief causes of sore throat are classified as follows:

1. **Traumatic**
   (a) foreign bodies (fish bones)
   (b) irritant fluids (alcohol)

    (c) overheated food and drink
    (d) smoking
    (e) inadequate air conditioning (associated with mouth-breathing)
    (f) industrial fumes
    (g) associated gastric reflux

2. **Inflammatory**
    (a) acute and chronic pharyngitis
    (b) acute and chronic tonsillitis
    (c) secondary to sinus infection
    (d) aphthous ulceration
    (e) herpetic ulceration (Ramsay Hunt).

3. **Neoplastic**
    (a) ulcerated malignant tumours of
        (i) nasopharynx
        (ii) oropharynx
        (iii) base of tongue
        (iv) hypopharynx
        (v) paralaryngeal region

4. **Others**
    (a) glossopharyngeal neuralgia
    (b) elongated styloid process

14. Hoarseness

Hoarseness and other alternations in voice production are usually due to structural changes in the vocal cord which impair its ability to vibrate. Less often, diseases which affect the tension and movements of the cord or the expiratory blast may be responsible. Voice change is common enough in all age groups and although, in the majority, it is due to benign self-limiting conditions, the importance of the rule that **hoarseness in the adult must always be considered indicative of malignancy until it can be proven otherwise** cannot be overemphasized.

The diagnosis cannot be made without mirror examination of the larynx and, indeed, direct examination under anaesthesia will often be necessary to reach a final decision as to the exact nature of the cause. This will always require referral to an ENT department. Nevertheless, much presumptive evidence regarding the likely aetiology and appropriate preliminary treatment can be obtained by intelligent history-taking.

HOARSENESS OF RECENT ONSET

In children, inflammation of the vocal cords as part of an upper respiratory infection is usually responsible: multiple papillomatosis of the vocal cords due to virus infection is a rare cause. Malignant lesions in the young are practically unknown.

The cause of hoarseness of recent onset in adults may be obvious from a history of prior upper respiratory infection leading to inflammatory swelling of the vocal cords and as such can safely be treated expectantly with the essential proviso that if it does not recover in one month a specialist opinion will be sought.

Treatment of persistent nasal and pharyngeal infection with antibiotics, decongestants, and inhalations, coupled with voice rest and restriction of tobacco and inhalations, will usually be sufficient to restore normal function. Concomitant sinusitis and pulmonary disease (including tuberculosis) should always be sought for and treated as necessary.

CHRONIC HOARSENESS

The main diagnostic therapeutic problems arise when the symptom is of longer standing — again the history may provide helpful guides as to the cause. Children are usually chronically hoarse because of vocal abuse — many of them shout and scream. Those who use their voices professionally — teachers and singers, especially if there has been no formal training in voice production — and those who work in loud noise, are particularly susceptible to chronic laryngitis and heavy consumption of alcohol and tobacco are often aggravating factors.

The causes of chronic hoarseness include:

1. **Local.** Loss of the smooth, sharp edge of the vocal cord due to inflammation, polyps, infiltration by mucopolysaccharide in hypothyroidism, fibrous nodes, leukoplakia, papillomata, and carcinoma.

2. **Neurological.** Impairment of the movement or tension in one or both vocal cords. These occur in recurrent nerve paralysis, myasthenia gravis, and Parkinsonism.

3. **General.** Weakness of the expiratory blast due to compression of the trachea or general weakness.

Local causes

Treatment

When mirror examination indicates chronic inflammation or a limited benign lesion, voice rest and the avoidance of perpetuating factors may be all that is required. If there is any uncertainty about the diagnosis, then direct examination with the operating microscope under general anaesthesia is essential so that the nature of the disease can be assessed precisely and abnormal tissue removed for histological examination.

The removal of polypi and nodes must be followed by speech therapy to correct the abnormal method of voice production which was responsible for the disease in the first place.

If carcinoma is confirmed by histological examination the method of treatment depends on the *extent* of the disease. Lesions limited to the vocal cord itself usually respond to radiotherapy. When there is involvement of paralaryngeal tissues with impairment of cord mobility or palpable spread to the deep cervical glands, although the reponse to deep X-ray may be tried, usually radical surgery comprising total laryngectomy with dissection of the neck glands combined with radiotherapy is required (Figs. 33 and 34). The prognosis is related to the extent of the disease, lesions limited to the vocal cord do best (85% five-year cure) but overall there is only a 50% five-year survival following laryngectomy. Many patients can be partially rehabilitated by learning oesophageal speech, a technique of communication in which swallowed air is belched from the oesophagus and formulated into meaningful sounds in the pharynx and mouth.

Neurological and neoplastic causes

A less common disturbance of voice production is vocal cord **paralysis** due to lesions of the vagus nerve which through its recurrent and superior laryngeal branches innervates the intrinsic muscles of the larynx. From above downwards these are:

1. Lesions near the jugular foramen usually with progressive involvement of the ninth, eleventh, and twelfth cranial nerves.
    (a) Tumours of the posterior cranial fossa such as meningioma, neuroma, and glomus jugulare.
    (b) Tumours of the nasopharynx such as carcinoma, mixed salivary tumour, and reticulosarcoma.
2. Lesions in the neck.
    (a) Tumours of the vagus nerve — neurilemminoma.
    (b) Carcinoma of the larynx.
    (c) Carcinoma of the hypopharynx, oesophagus, and thyroid.
    (d) Malignant cervical lymph nodes.
    (e) Surgical trauma during thyroidectomy, excision of pharyngeal pouch, and tracheostomy.
    (f) Penetrating wounds.

3. Lesions in the mediastinum (left recurrent laryngeal nerve only).
    (a) Carcinoma of the bronchus (very frequent) and the apex of the lung (Pancoast syndrome).
    (b) Carcinoma of the oesophagus.
    (c) Malignant lymph nodes and lymphatic tumours.
    (d) Cardiac enlargement and cardiac surgery.
    (e) Aortic aneurysm.
    (f) Peripheral neuritis.
    (g) Penetrating knife and gunshot wounds.

Finally, there is a small group of patients in whom, as a result of psychiatric disease, usually hysteria, there is total loss or weakness of the voice. Such a patient can usually cough loudly but produces only a whisper when asked to speak.

In conclusion, the importance of a high index of suspicion that hoarseness persisting for more than one month has a sinister connotation is stressed.

REVISION: THE CAUSES OF HOARSENESS

For revision purposes, the chief causes of hoarseness are classified as follows:

1. **Traumatic**
   (a) blunt and penetrating injuries to the larynx and its motor nerve supply
   (b) excessive use of tobacco and alcohol
   (c) industrial fumes
   (d) incorrect voice production
   (e) aortic aneurysm

2. **Inflammatory**
   (a) acute and chronic non-specific inflammation often secondary to sinus or pulmonary infection
   (b) when chronic, may result in generalized mucosal thickening (pachydermia)
   (c) specific infections (tuberculosis and syphilis)

3. **Neoplastic**
   (a) benign
      (i) papillomata (multiple in children)
      (ii) fibroma (singers' nodes)
      (iii) polypi (chronic trauma)
      (iv) chondroma
      (v) angioma
   (b) Malignant — squamous carcinoma

4. **Neurological**
   Penetrating injury or pressure and involvement with swellings arising along the route of the vagus nerve and its recurrent laryngeal branch. Note that because of its longer course, the left nerve is the more often affected.

5. **Others**
   (a) localized thickening from precancerous lesions (leukoplakia)
   (b) generalized thickening in hypothyroidism

15. Lumps in the neck

In this area of ENT diseases, more than in any other, the history is often of only limited assistance in reaching a diagnosis. Of course, there are exceptions — for example, when a soft translucent supraclavicular mass has been present from birth it will almost certainly prove to be a cystic hygroma. Again, a tender mass behind the angle of the mandible during the course of acute tonsillitis in a child is more than likely to be due to inflammatory lymphadenopathy.

However, the patient's age and general state of health, the time since the swelling was first noticed, the presence of tenderness or pain, continued enlargement, and possibly associated symptoms in the throat or elsewhere may all prove valuable guides towards a diagnosis.

Causes

For practical purposes, the main causes of swellings in the neck can best be classified anatomically in regard to the various structures from which they arise (Fig. 34).

The overwhelming majority of lumps in the neck arising **laterally** are due to inflammatory or neoplastic disease of the **cervical lymph nodes.** Of the inflammatory causes, recurrent tonsillitis during the **first decade** accounts for most and the jugulodigastric glands may be palpable for one or two years after the cessation of recurrent tonsillitis. In this situation the glands themselves do not require specific treatment and the tonsils should be treated on their merits as previously indicated.

In patients **aged 40 years or more,** a malignant cause (primary or secondary) must be suspected until proven otherwise.

The incidence of **tuberculous adenitis** has been considerably reduced by pasteurization of milk and the control of phthisis. Nevertheless, isolated cases do occur usually in the young and, again, the diagnosis is based on a high index of suspicion, a history of exposure to infected milk or a person suffering from open pulmonary tuberculosis. Confirmation is histological and bacteriological retrospectively after excision. Tuberculous adenitis is to be differentiated from **branchial cyst** which is soft and transluminant.

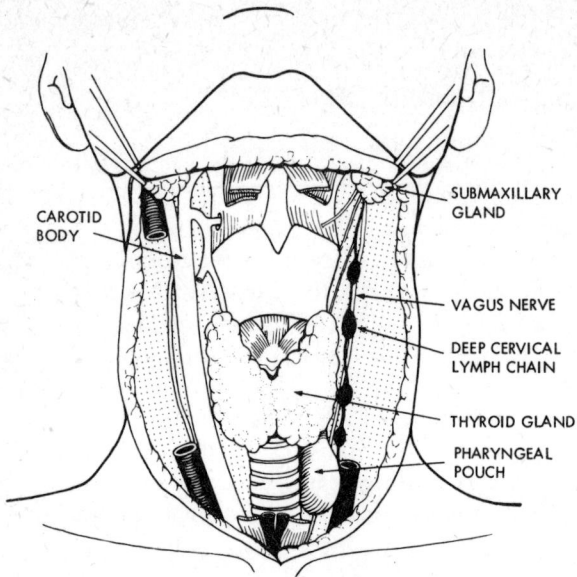

CAROTID
BODY

SUBMAXILLARY
GLAND

VAGUS NERVE

DEEP CERVICAL
LYMPH CHAIN

THYROID GLAND

PHARYNGEAL
POUCH

Fig. 34.

Glandular fever (infective mononucleosis) causes generalized cervical glandular swellings and in this the diagnosis is suggested by its association with acute inflammation of the tonsils which are frequently covered with patches of white membrane, and confirmed by blood examination for atypical mononucleocytes and serology (Paul–Bunnell test).

The infectious fevers of childhood are accompanied by enlargement of the cervical glands — those of the posterior triangle are characteristically most affected in **rubella.**

Neoplastic diseases of the lymphatic system may present with cervical adenopathy. The most common of these are Hodgkin's disease, the reticuloses, and leukaemia. In the first two, excision of a gland, marrow biopsy, and chest X-ray may be necessary to establish the diagnosis and treatment will be by radiotherapy and/or chemotherapy. Peripheral blood films and the presence of lymphadenopathy elsewhere will confirm leukaemic disease.

Enlargement of the cervical glands may be due to **metastatic spread from a pharyngeal or laryngeal malignancy.** Because excision of a gland for biopsy in such cases may prejudice future management severely by cutting across lines of lymphatic drainage and disseminating malignant cells, every attempt to identify the primary tumour must be made *before* treatment is started. The vital importance of a full examination of all the possible sites of a carcinomatous or adenocarcinomatous primary lesion in the naso-pharynx, base of the tongue, oropharynx, larynx, laryngopharynx, oesophagus, thyroid, and lungs, and elsewhere, e.g. kidney, pro-state, and stomach, augmented by lateral X-rays of the neck and, if necessary, by radiological studies, cannot be overemphasized in the evaluation of all patients presenting with a cervical lump. **(It is bad practice to perform excisional biopsy before the possi-bility of an ENT primary has been excluded.)**

Treatment

Although localized malignant disease of the pharynx and larynx can frequently be cured by radiotherapy, this is rarely possible once the tumour has spread to the cervical lymphatics. Glandular involvement is usually an indication for combined surgery and radiotherapy, with wide removal of the primary lesion in continuity with the deep cervical lymph nodes. The fact that laryngectomy and laryngopharyngectomy are essentially grossly mutilating opera-tions, are frequently only palliative, and provide a five-year survival for no more than 50% of patients, emphasizes the importance of early diagnosis and carefully planned management in all cases of malignant lymphadenopathy.

Diffuse, often fluctuant **swellings,** nowadays seen only rarely, are usually inflammatory extensions along the tissue planes of the neck from the mastoid (Bezold's abscess), the floor of the mouth (Ludwig's angina), from the laryngeal cartilages (parichondritis), and from the pharyngeal wall (parapharyngeal abscess). Their diagnosis is based on identifying the primary lesion and treating this on its merits, usually with antibiotics and by drainage of pus when appropriate.

Swellings of the salivary glands may be inflammatory, due to viral (mumps) or bacterial infection (in the submandibular gland, often associated with a calculus in the duct), or neoplastic. The majority of tumours are potentially or frankly malignant and include mixed salivary tumours, cylindroma, adenocarcinoma, and squamous cell carcinoma. Bacterial infection will usually respond to antibiotic therapy but, if recurrent, excision of the gland may be necessary; tumours require total excision.

Although **medial swellings** may be due to the spread of infection from elsewhere (see below), they are more often thyroid in origin and take the form of either a generalized enlargement such as in goitre, or a localized adenoma. A medial swelling, often recurrently inflamed, situated close to the body of hyoid is practically always a thyroglossal cyst. The treatment of these swellings is based on tests of thyroid function and is usually primary medical but may also be surgical and radiotherapeutic if malignancy is confirmed.

Laryngeal and pharyngeal pouches cause swellings close to the midline and may give rise to vocal symptoms or dysphagia. They are usually diagnosed radiologically and by direct examination under anaesthesia. Treatment is by excision.

Neurolemminoma of the tenth cranial nerve occurs rarely as a firm unilateral mass in the anterior cervical triangle and requires excision. The diagnosis is based on its situation and presentation and confirmed by histological examination

Carotid body tumours, arising from the carotid body at the bifurcation of the common carotid artery, may be associated with fluctuating hypertension and occasionally concomitant glomus jugulare tumours. Their diagnosis is based on their characteristic situation, pulsatile nature, and angiography. Their treatment requires considerable clinical judgement. The removal of large carotid body tumours necessitates grafting the carotid artery and carries a high risk of hemiplegia.

16. Airway obstruction

Obstruction to breathing arising from causes in the pharynx and larynx usually develops rapidly and is one of the most acute life-threatening emergencies which occur in ENT practice. Its solution depends on a proper understanding of the causes of asphyxia and their management.

Causes

Lesions which obstruct the passage of air to the lungs can be classified as (1) due to external compression, (2) arising within the walls of the airway, and (3) occurring within the lumen (Fig. 35).

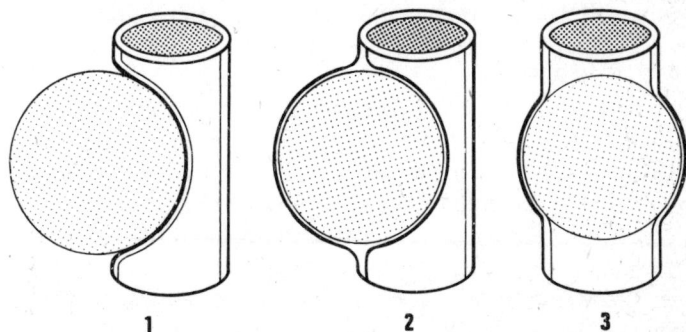

Fig. 35. Tracheal obstruction can be caused by (1) extramural, (2) intramural, and (3) intraluminal masses.

Causes compressing the airway from outside
Because of the arrangement of fascial planes in the neck, blood, pus, and air arising from inflammation and trauma to other areas can track to, accumulate around, and rapidly compress the airway and demand urgent relief. Compression from neoplastic masses in the neck such as thyroid carcinoma, will usually occur more slowly.

Causes arising from the walls of the airway
   (a) Commonly, acute airway obstruction may arise directly from swelling of the pharyngeal and laryngeal tissues due to inflammation or neoplasia.

In young children, inflammatory swelling may complicate acute pharyngitis (croup) and is especially acute and characteristically dangerous when epiglottic swelling due to haemophilis influenzae infection obstructs the supralaryngeal region (epiglottiditis).

(b) In older patients, as a rule, airway embarrassment develops more slowly. Involvement of the vocal cords or paralaryngeal structures by squamous carcinoma is the most frequent cause.

Causes within the lumen

These are invariably foreign bodies, usually affect the very young, and are fatal unless treated immediately with determination. Children can inhale practically any object small enough to pass the pillars of the tonsil. Should a foreign body lodge above or between the vocal cords, only, (a) its immediate displacement manually or by upending the child and forcibly striking the back, or (b) laryngotomy, can prevent immediate death from asphyxiation.

Clinical presentation

The asphyxiating patient is breathless, cyanotic, and distressed.

Differentiation between laryngeal obstruction and pulmonary insufficiency is based on a history and the results of chest examination which will indicate pneumonic disease on one hand and, on the other, a history of pharyngeal or laryngeal disease or foreign body coupled with an inability to expand the lungs as indicated by violent action of the accessory muscles of respiration with indrawing of the supraclavicular and intercostal spaces. In laryngeal obstruction, deterioration will usually proceed quite rapidly, with increasing cyanosis, stridor, and weakness, to collapse and death.

Treatment

The patient's survival depends entirely upon immediate diagnosis and prompt re-establishment of the airway.

In **young children** suffering from croupy laryngeal oedema, steam inhalations, intramuscular antibiotic, and oral decongestants (Actifed Compound Linctus — triprolidine hydrochloride pseudoephedrine hydrochloride, codeine phosphate), steroids, and sedation (Phenergan Elixir — promethazine hydrochloride), will usually provide a rapid remission. If such a remission is not obviously forthcoming then epiglotiditis should be presumed and treated with the utmost energy and promptitude by immediate admission to a respiratory failure unit. Direct laryngoscopy under anaesthesia will demonstrate the site and nature of the obstruction, allow the removal of any foreign body, and permit intubation. Once the immediate danger has been overcome, further treatment with humidification, ampicillin, steroids, and decongestants will reduce the inflammatory state until detubation can be performed with safety — usually within a few days.

When facilities for intubation are not immediately available, then laryngotomy with a wide-bore needle forced through the space between the anterior borders of the thyroid and cricoid cartilages will be urgently required, and should be performed at once, before the development of terminal respiratory depression which inexorably follows prolonged anoxia. Once the airway has been re-established in this way, tracheotomy (Fig. 36) or intubation can be performed to gain reliable control of the airway.

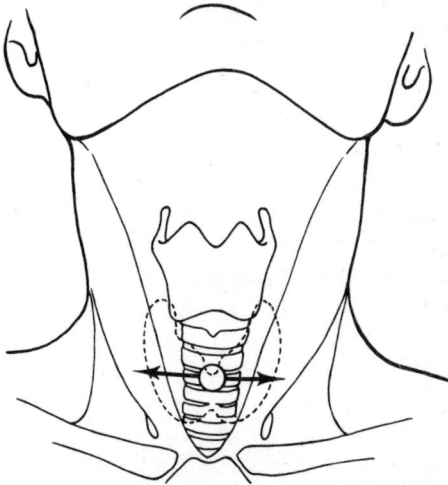

Fig. 36. Tracheotomy — using a horizontal skin incision, after dividing the thyroid isthmus between clamps the trachea is opened by cutting a hole through the third and fourth tracheal rings and removing part of one ring. The airway is then maintained with a silver or plastic tracheostomy tube.

Once the airway has been re-established, the management of the underlying disease can then proceed.

In summary, when there is acute airway obstruction, management should be as follows:

1. Assess the situation and the condition of the patient as regards the degree of urgency.

2. Inspect the airway to locate the nature and level of obstruction.

3. Remove a foreign body, if possible.

4. If the obstructing lesion is not removable or is not rapidly responsive to medication such as with steroids and antibiotics, then bypass it

    (a) internally by oropharyngeal or nasopharyngeal intubation,
       or

    (b) externally by

        (i) laryngotomy in an acute emergency, or

        (ii) tracheostomy as an elective procedure.

In patients whose respiratory obstruction is due to malignant involvement of the larynx or trachea, such as from carcinoma of the larynx, postcricoid region, or the thyroid gland, progress is usually less rapid than in the inflammatory conditions which affect young children.

The management of such conditions requires careful judgement and is decided on by the extent and nature of the lesion. In tumours which are amenable to surgical treatment, radical excision should be carried out as soon as practicable. In cases of more extensive disease, tracheotomy may be indicated either as palliation or as a preliminary to treatment with radiotherapy.

17. Dysphagia

Excluding obstructions of the throat by foreign bodies (which occur at any age), dysphagia is predominantly a symptom of middle and later life. Dysphagia, or difficulty in swallowing, is due to pain or obstruction, or both.

Painful causes

1. Inflammation of mucosa and lymph tissue due to trauma, foreign bodies, or acute infection.
2. Secondary inflammation and ulceration of neoplasms.
3. Chemical irritation from ingested fluids.

Obstructive causes

1. Neuromuscular incoordination which results in crico-pharyngeal spasm and which occurs in conjunction with hiatus hernia or incompetence of the lower oesophageal sphincter.
2. Swelling arising from the tissues of the throat, such as tumours (usually malignant) of the postcricoid region and the oesophagus, pouches, and diverticulae formed by outward herniation of the mucosa into the tissues of the neck or thorax.
3. Swellings of nearby structures which obliterate the lumen by pressure from without such as thyroid tumours, lymphomata, and malignant glands in the neck or at the hilum of the lung.

Clinical presentation

The onset of dysphagia is rarely acute and although the patient may eventually present as an emergency because food has occluded a narrowed lumen, there is usually a history of recent and persistent difficulty in swallowing solid food or tablets.

Total inability to swallow anything, including saliva, is strongly suggestive of a malignant cause or foreign body. When the latter is responsible, the patient will usually say so and its location will be confirmed by X-ray using contrast studies if the object is not radio-opaque.

When malignancy causes dysphagia, the patient's pale, emaciated appearance will suggest the cause early in the course of the disease.

When dysphagia is not total, then the diagnosis of painful causes usually presents little difficulty. The pyrexic patient will describe his developing symptoms of upper respiratory infection and the cause of pain will be apparent on inspecting the throat. By contrast, the patient who has swallowed caustic or acid by accident or by design will be pale, clammy, and shocked, and his burnt lips and palate and the contents of a nearby bottle will confirm the diagnosis.

Patients whose dysphagia is the result of cricopharyngeal spasm because of neuromuscular incoordination do not usually appear ill, although they may be pale because of anaemia, are usually over-weight, and often female with a history of dysphagia dating back to their last pregnancy. They complain of feeling a lump in the throat or of the need to force food past an obstruction which they localize at cricoid level, occupying one to two seconds after initiating the act of swallowing. They often suffer from 'heartburn' especially at night.

Because these symptoms are similar to those of both pharyngeal pouch and early postcricoid carcinoma, it is essential that these patients be fully investigated radiologically and, if necessary, by endoscopy to establish the correct diagnosis.

When the cause is extraluminal, straight X-rays and radiological contrast studies will demonstrate the site and cause of dysphagia. Mediastinal masses are usually neoplastic and thoracotomy and biopsy are necessary to establish the exact diagnosis.

Treatment

1. Acute tonsillitis and quinsy will be treated with antibiotics, etc. as previously indicated.

2. Corrosive burns are treated in hospital as a matter of great urgency by
   (a) neutralization with the appropriate agent,
   (b) endoscopy to identify the site and extent of damage,
   (c) broad-spectrum antibiotic combined with steroid to reduce scarring and subsequent stenosis.

3. Cricopharyngeal spasm and hiatus hernia are treated with antacids such as Asilone (dimethicone, dried aluminium hydroxide gel, sorbitol), Gastrocote (alginic acid, dried aluminium hydroxide gel, trisilicate, sodium bicarbonate), and Gaviscon (alginic acid, magnesium trisilicate, dried aluminium hydroxide gel, sodium

bicarbonate) and with various cholinergic agents. Weight reduction and elevation of the bed head are usually recommended. Large hernias may require surgical treatment. Mucosal webs at the cricopharynx will require endoscopic dilatation.

4. The treatment of the malignant lesions of the pharynx is described in Chapter 13. Carcinoma of the öesophagus has a very poor prognosis but some palliation is often possible with radio-therapy and swallowing can be maintained temporarily by means of an intraluminal tube. Eventually, a gastrostomy will be required.

Malignant masses in the mediastinum are usually treated with a combination of deep X-ray and cytotoxic therapy, whose value is again largely palliative.

18. Foreign bodies in the ear, nose, and throat

Foreign bodies of the ENT region can frequently lead to the serious consequences of airway obstruction and sepsis. Their removal is often a difficult matter because of inaccessibility and the very nature of the object itself.

As a rule, in young children, the diagnosis is not always obvious because the foreign body is either self-administered — and children do not always willingly admit their folly — or inhaled by those too young to co-operate as historians. In older patients in whom foreign bodies consist of objects such as swallowed bones or dentures, the history is usually helpful and relevant to the outcome.

THE EAR

Although foreign bodies in the external auditory meatus are frequently asymptomatic they often give rise to chronic infection causing discomfort, pain, discharge, and hearing loss. Although water-resistant objects can usually be removed by syringing, as a rule; especially when they are hygroscopic, they should be removed under direct vision with a hooked probe. In the absence of cooperation, which is usual when there is inflammation, general anaesthesia is mandatory. Care should be taken to avoid displacing the foreign body past the constricted bottle-neck junction which exists where the cartilaginous and osseous canal walls unite.

Although cerumen (wax) is not a foreign body in the strict sense it is removed in a similar way by syringing. The success of this procedure is often enhanced by prior softening with oily drops. When exostoses (bony nodules arising from the walls of the ear canal) are present, the removal of wax from their medial aspect may require to be carried out under general anaesthesia.

THE NOSE

Foreign bodies in the nose can pose a sinister threat in that at any time either spontaneously or during their attempted removal, they may be displaced into the larynx and cause asphyxia. Undetected, they are invariably complicated by infection and are undoubtedly the commonest cause of **unilateral** purulent blood-stained and foul-smelling nasal discharge in the young. They should be removed with a hook under direct vision using local anaesthetic drops, or if the child is uncooperative, under general anaesthesia.

THE THROAT

Inhaled foreign bodies in the very young may be rapidly fatal if they lodge in or immediately above the larynx. Rapidly developing cyanosis and respiratory distress without other obvious cause will strongly suggest the cause which will require urgent and determined action for its solution. Immediate facilities for tracheotomy are highly unlikely and prompt upending of the child with forcible blows applied to the back may dislodge the foreign body. Otherwise, immediate laryngotomy is essential to prevent death from asphyxia.

Inhaled foreign bodies which pass through the larynx usually become lodged in the right main bronchus. If an adult was present, then the diagnosis will be suggested by his evidence that the child had been playing with some small object (which later could not be found), choked and coughed, became a 'bad colour' which somewhat improved, and proceeded to become increasingly breathless, distressed, and restless. Frequently, with infants suffering recurrent attacks of 'bronchitis', there is no history of foreign body but a chest X-ray will demonstrate an area of pulmonary collapse and the object itself, if it is radio-opaque.

Peanuts, because of their tendency to swell and cause inflammation, require urgent removal.

Removal of a foreign body can usually be carried out by bronchoscopy under general anaesthesia, but small hard angulated objects may require thoracotomy.

Swallowed foreign bodies are essentially the preserve of the edentulous adult although, of course, the problem does occasionally arise in children too. Fish and meat bones can easily pass the palate whose sensation is reduced by a dental plate or dulled by alcohol, and become lodged at the junction between the hypopharynx and oesophagus (cricopharyngeal sphincter). Badly fitting dentures can behave likewise. X-ray and, if necessary, barium studies will usually indicate the location of the foreign body which should be removed by oesophagoscopy under general anaesthesia. Because injury of the pharyngeal or oesophageal wall by sharp foreign bodies is common and will result in dangerous complications which include cervical abscess, mediastinitis, and erosion of a large vessel, removal of the foreign body should be arranged promptly.

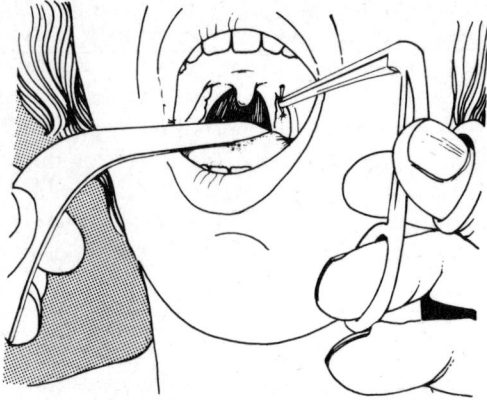

Fig. 37.

Of less danger are small fish bones which frequently become stuck in one of the crypts of the palatal or lingual tonsil. The patient often locates the object with fair accuracy and if a careful search of these areas is made, using full illumination with a tongue spatula, the bone can often be extracted with forceps without recourse to general anaesthesia (Fig. 37).

Index